Dalia _____ _____ovitch-Weiss

Producer & International Distributor
eBookPro Publishing
www.ebook-pro.com

A Child Without a Shadow
Dalia Harel, Ela Moscovitch-Weiss

Contact: harel_sh@netvision.net.il
ISBN 9798521000951

A CHILD WITHOUT A SHADOW

PROFESSOR SHAUL HAREL
A Story of Resilience

DALIA HAREL
ELA MOSCOVITCH-WEISS

Contents

PREFACE BY
PROFESSOR JOHN R. BENFIELD, MD, FACS

The importance of this book transcends the obvious. The apparent and very real significance is the survival of four-year-old Charlie Hilsberg of Brussels because *Mademoiselle,* a 20-year-old gentile beauty, heroically stepped forward and arranged his becoming a hidden child. The Germans murdered his parents, his brother and his sister, and six million other Jews. After his time as a hidden child, Charlie learned to smile and laugh again, made his way to Israel, and became Shaul Harel when Ben Gurion said every Israeli needs an Israeli name. Shaul married Dalia, an outstanding Sabra. While he pioneered in pediatric neurology, tirelessly and most effectively, he kept his story as a hidden child much to himself, at least insofar as the Harel children were concerned. This was perhaps analogous to the fact that most soldiers who have survived the horrors of active battle tend to keep that awful experience to themselves. Shaul's eventual decision to tell his tale, and to take his children back to Brussels is wonderful. The world has benefitted from the documentary that was filmed, and the songs that he has created, and from this book.

In my view, even greater than the obvious in Professor Harel's tale, is told by him in his book when he describes his thoughts and sentiments during his presidency of the world's leading professional organization in his specialty. That year, the group met near Auschwitz. He was near Hitler's worst death camp, and as president he had the authority to grant or to decline a German colleague's permission to speak. At that moment, he recalled his parents who had been murdered in Auschwitz, and how they would have savored the moment when Shaul ruled over the German in his group.

In part, the additional message of Professor Harel's story is illustrated by Yad Vashem in Jerusalem, and the Museum of the Jewish People in Tel Aviv. The former describes the inhumane brutality of the Holocaust in the 1930s and 1940s. The latter tells of 5,781 years of survival of the Jewish People, despite recurrent and persistent anti-Semitism, persecution and murder. The transition of Charlie Hilsberg of Brussels into Professor Shaul Harel of Tel Aviv is a shining, stirring example of Jewish resilience and adaptability.

Why am I privileged to write about this book? I was born in Vienna as Hans Bienenfeld. Now I am a past president of the Society of Thoracic Surgeons, the largest and most influential group in my specialty. Shaul and I bonded immediately when we met about 15 years ago. I consider him like a brother. Yet, our backgrounds are different. My father, mother and I had the good fortune to escape the Holocaust by becoming refugees in New York City. Our view of the present is the same. Shaul and I share our commitment to teaching young Jews and gentiles alike about the incredible, admirable adaptability and resilience of the Jewish people.

John R. Benfield, MD, FACS
Professor of Surgery Emeritus
David Geffen School of Medicine at UCLA
Los Angeles, California
j.benfield@ucla.edu
(310) 889-9186
(310) 413-3704 (mobile)

DEDICATION

This book is dedicated first and foremost to my parents, Moshe and Perla, to my sister Tola, and to my brother Marcel, from whom I was torn away when I was five, and who were later murdered in the Auschwitz extermination camp. Unfortunately, I have only vague memories of them. From what I've been told, they were modest, warm and brave, and I'm sure that the love in which they enveloped me as a child allowed me to successfully deal with the hardships that I was dealt in the years that followed. This book is intended to commemorate them.

This book is dedicated to my brother Israel and my sister, Regina, who were there for me after World War II ended, and it is thanks to them that I immigrated to Israel. They cushioned my life with concern and love, formed a supportive family and gave me solid support.

This book is dedicated to the brave rescue team that saved Jewish children in Belgium, and to Ida Sterno and Andree Geulen in particular, who took me from my parents' home and kept me hidden throughout the war. Of all of them, only Andree Geulen survived, and thanks to her, when I was close to 70 years old, I learned about my wandering path during the war and about her important part in returning me to my family and people.

This book is also dedicated to the counselors at the orphanage in Lasne, Siegi Hirsch, the first person after the war to make me feel joy again and to put a smile on my face. He did the same for the other hidden children, who, over time, became my friends, such as Robert Fuks.

And naturally, this book is also dedicated to my immediate family—to my wife Dalia, who has been my partner all these years and allowed me to devote a significant part of my time to medical work; to my beloved children, who brought light into our lives, Tali, Ronit and Gili; and to my beloved grand-children, Idan, Noya, Inbar, Ofir, Ido, Liam and Mia, who continue to fill our lives with hope and optimism.

And finally, I dedicate this book to all those principals, teachers, advisors, co-workers, lifelong friends and the long list of the dedicated staff who worked with me at the Sourasky Medical Center in Tel Aviv, allowing me to fulfill my dreams.

PROLOGUE—LJUBLJANA 1998

Of all his achievements in pediatric neurology and child development, of all the awards that he received, the ceremonies that he attended and the lectures that he gave, Professor Shaul Harel had never felt greater satisfaction than he did at that moment.

It happened in the fall of 1998 in Ljubljana, Slovenia. He had just been elected president of the International Child Neurology Association and convened a meeting of the association's executive board. He sat at the head of the table and looked at the raised hand of the German representative, who was asking for his permission to speak. His gaze lingered on the German representative's face, and for one moment, he wondered if the man's father or grandfather had been one of those officers who had burst into his parents' home in Brussels one day and forcibly removed them, then sent them on Transport No. 20 to Auschwitz and to their horrifying death.

Who would have believed that the very same child who had been forced to hide from the Germans during World War II, whose lives was put in danger and was almost considered lost, would be sitting such and such years later at the head of that table; that representatives from all over the world would be asking him for the right to speak so that he could hear their professional opinions? If only his parents could see him.

With a polite nod, and with the ironic restraint he had acquired, Prof. Harel gave the German representative permission to speak.

THE FAMILY, THE "EXODUS" TO FRANCE, THE HOLOCAUST IN BELGIUM

WARSAW 1926-1932

One winter evening in 1926, Idel Hilsberg stroked his well-groomed black beard, and looked out the window at the men and women strolling down the sidewalk on Majzelsa Street in his beloved city, Warsaw.

From where he was standing, he could see people coming and going from Itche Parnas' liquor store. Itche was the mohel, and he'd circumcised all of Idel's sons. He noticed the bachelors on their way home from work stopping for a meal at Leiser's restaurant—that is, if they weren't tempted a few feet before to order pepper-spiced peas with a mug of beer on the side from Treitel's stand. The street was quiet and there was no trace of the demonstration that the Communist party had held the day before.

He looked at the many pedestrians and thought with concern about the strange ways of fate and about what was still in store for his son, Moshe, and his three grandchildren. He admitted to himself that of all his children, he felt most connected to Moshe. Perhaps it was because of his sensitive and doleful eyes that looked at the world through the thin frames of his round glasses. Maybe it was his deep voice, the pleasant singing voice of a cantor, or because of the deep compassion that he felt in his heart for his son, who had just recently been widowed and was left on his own to care for three young children. He thought affectionately about seven-year-old Tola, five-year-old Israel and two-year-old Marcel and wondered how the children would grow up without a loving mother.

How relieved and happy he was when less than a year later, a match was found for his son, the gentle and kind-hearted Perla Rotblat, and he proposed to her.

Although she was three years his senior, Moshe felt that she was the woman who could fill his first wife's place and be a loving mother to his orphaned children.

Perla was from a wealthy and respected family from Warsaw's Jewish community. The family had lost its wealth due to the ravages of World War I. She was an attractive woman in her mid-thirties and still single. She had rejected all her suitors when she was younger because for many years, she had to take care of her ailing parents who, as mentioned, had lost all their wealth. Perla was not at all bitter and never felt like a victim. Perhaps that was why, as compensation for those lost years, at the then-considered grand old age of thirty-five, she was given a ready-made family: a husband with three children who desperately needed her.

She wholeheartedly devoted herself to those children as if they were her own, and they were soon calling her "Mama."

Although they had met through a matchmaker, it was impossible not to be impressed by the deep love that sparked between the couple. In private and with an awkward laugh that didn't suit his age, Moshe whispered to his mother, Shosha, that he felt as if he'd been hit by lightning when he saw Perla for the first time.

However, in Warsaw of the early 1930s, not everything seemed to be as romantic and promising. Anti-Semitism, a weed that had always been there waiting for the right climatic conditions in order to spread, managed to creep into many places with the help of the government's antisemitic policy. Even before the pogroms that would occur between 1934 and 1936, the repulsion and aversion felt toward Jews was obvious, with the limited positions they were permitted to have and with the small number of Jews accepted to universities. Even then, in another humiliating act, the Jewish students had to sit only on the left side of the lecture hall. The Jewish community lived with a constant and ominous sense of persecution.

Miras, Perla's younger sister, had immigrated to Brussels back in the 1920s. Miras' husband, who manufactured buttons, had quickly achieved financial success, and she wrote to Perla about that wonderful place, Belgium. Moshe's friend Mr. Kremer had also emigrated from Poland and owned a tie factory, and he invited Moshe to join him.

And so, in 1932, when Regina, the first child that Moshe and Perla had together, celebrated her fourth birthday, the couple decided that they, too, would emigrate to Belgium and settle in Brussels. Moshe, a diligent crafts-man whose father made ties, believed that ties would be in demand in every civilized place, and Western Europe, he claimed, was such a place. What was happening now in Warsaw in Poland would never happen in Belgium or France, he thought. The Hilsberg family packed up their belongings and moved, first to Antwerp and a year later to Brussels. They joined the growing stream of refugees from Eastern Europe who made it to Belgium, a relatively welcoming country between the two world wars. The refugees slowly became the majority of the Jewish community in Belgium. Although they didn't have Belgian citizenship, they were allowed to stay there with alien status. It didn't prevent them from becoming a community with well-developed public, po-litical and Jewish awareness, and they organized various areas of their life. First and foremost, they arranged mutual aid and help for refugees, as well as education, culture, sports, youth activities and more. All the movements that were active in the Jewish world—religious, Zionist, left-wing Zionist workers and communists—took root in the Jewish community in Belgium. Moshe Hilsberg, who loved to be active, also found his place there.

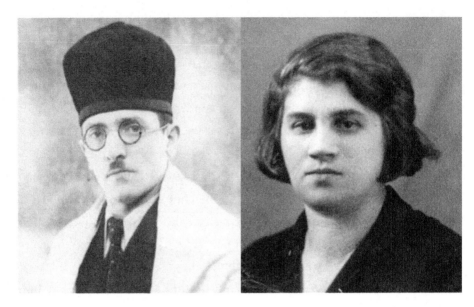

Moshe Hilsberg   Perla Hilsberg

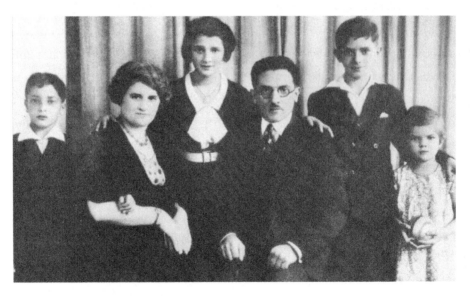

Family portrait taken after emigrating to Belgium. From left to right: Marcel, Perla, Tola, Moshe, Israel and Regina

BRUSSELS 1938

"Unfortunately," Joseph Schmidt was told as a young man, "despite your divine talent, you simply cannot appear before an audience."

This was not a case of anti-Semitism.

The last time that his height was measured, when his adolescence was over, the gifted singer's stature was about five feet. "That's why you won't be able to perform in operas," he was told; "but you will be able to record," he was immediately reassured.

Schmidt was a little bit discouraged, but he didn't give up. Over the years, he developed an international career and became known to everyone as one of the most famous Jewish cantors in Europe, a revered and popular opera and operetta singer, and he even starred in movies. His lyrical, tenor voice enchanted his listeners, and he did seem to grow a little taller, even if only from the strong admiration he received wherever he went during the 1920s and 30s, including Germany. Even Goebbels was a fan and gave orders to let him be.

It is easy to imagine, then, the astonishment and cries of joy that erupted from the mouths of the Hilsberg family when one Friday, Moshe Hilsberg, the father of the family, arrived home arm-in-arm with the singer from Czernowitz. The first thing that Joseph saw when he entered his new acquaintance's home was the beautiful face of nineteen-year-old Tola. Joseph Schmidt had a weakness not only for the aesthetics of music, but also for true beauty wherever it may be. He gave the young woman fervid glances before making an explicit proposal to her father, asking for her hand in marriage. Tola was embarrassed and ran to her room. He was a head shorter and fifteen years older than her, nothing like she'd imagined the man that she'd love.

Moshe smiled softly at Joseph and carefully explained to him that it wasn't really appropriate. Moshe was very disheartened and disappointed.

His disappointment, however, did not last long, as word of the world-renowned singer and cantor's visit had spread through the neighborhood and Moshe's Jewish neighbors, friends and acquaintances flocked to the inviting apartment at 37a Montenegro Street in the Saint-Gilles district to see him with their own two eyes.

Schmidt took the fuss he was causing in stride. He sat on the sofa in the living room, his feet barely touching the floor, and invited Moshe, who also had a good singing voice, to join him in a song.

The family was not ultra-religious, but Moshe was the cantor at the small neighborhood synagogue, or *shtiebel* as they called it in Yiddish, and he would sing cantorial and folk songs in a beautiful, deep voice. They sang, unaware that the famous and esteemed Jewish tenor's life would end in 1942, before his thirty-eighth birthday, in a refugee camp in Switzerland, where he lay ill without medical attention after the American visa intended for him had been taken by someone else.

That evening, however, when none of them could even imagine the hardships to come, Moshe Hilsberg leaned back in his chair at the head of the table and looked lovingly at his wife Perla, who was serving challahs, gefilte fish and her famous roast in a velvety sauce with potatoes on the side. Friday evenings were his favorite time of the week when he welcomed the Sabbath. After saying Kiddush, he murmured a few personal words: "I thank you God for all the good you have given me—a lovely wife, wonderful children and a reasonable livelihood."

Moshe learned at a young age that the secret to happiness lies, among other things, in gratitude for what you receive and in being able to appreciate what you have. His heart had already been broken once, when his first wife suddenly passed away, leaving him a young widower with three children to look after, and he valued and cherished his second marriage to a woman he loved who gave him two more adorable children.

On that autumn evening in 1938, Moshe Hilsberg looked at his close, warm family, at his three older children—Tola, his eldest, who was a beautiful and bubbly girl and constantly surrounded by friends; Israel (Salek), who was an outstanding student and about to finish high school; and Marcel, with his angel face. Then he turned and looked at his younger two: ten-year-old, golden-haired Regina, and at Charles-David, or Charlie for short, the sweet one-year-old baby who arrived quite a few years after Regina. He came as a big surprise, when Charlie's mother was forty-five. Moshe remembered Charlie's bris, which was celebrated with great joy and merriment at the Adolphe Max restaurant in Brussels. All the leaders of the Jewish community in Brussels, and many others in the neighborhood, participated in the celebration because as the cantor, he was well-known, and he was liked in the community.

They lived in a modest but pleasant neighborhood, Saint Gilles, where many Jews of the lower class lived. Still, there were enough rooms for everyone in their second-floor rented apartment. The girls lived in one room: Tola and Regina, who were always sharing secrets; and Israel and Marcel, who were the greatest of friends in the other. The parents had the third room, where Charlie's crib stood, and they used the fourth for guests. The fifth room was used as a workshop for making ties, where the boys would help their father. The kitchen was small, but they all managed to cram in. Regina loved to reminisce over those days, and she used to say that they even had a special cabinet there for the Passover dishes, which she loved peeking into.

Their home was always a happy one. In the few remaining pictures that Regina had, their mother Perla's expression is slightly grave, but Regina remembers her as a warm, loving woman, working all day to take care of her husband and five children, occasionally mentioning how much she longed for her family in Poland.

Everyone called Charlie *"Chierkele,"* which is a small cloth duster in Yiddish, because he used to crawl between his parents', brothers' and sisters' legs all the time with a constant cheeky smile on his face. Charlie-Shaul's memories of his childhood were very vague, and he barely remembered his father and mother. The few images that are engraved in his memory are of visiting the synagogue with his father, who would wrap him in his tallit during prayers, and of his brother Marcel carrying him on his shoulders and running with him down their hallway at home. As the youngest, he was the pride and joy of the family, and his happy childhood must have given him the resilience he needed for the dark years that came later.

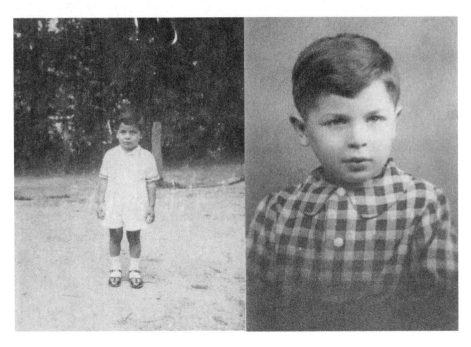

Charlie as a young boy

Moshe's face glowed with pleasure the evening that Joseph Schmidt was his guest at home. He thought it had been a wise move to leave Warsaw six years earlier, but he felt a twinge in his heart when he thought of his parents, for whom he felt an intense longing. His father, Idel, had a distinguished appearance and a black beard, and his mother, Shoshaleh, was a short and energetic woman. He thought about last Passover when he said goodbye to his parents. In 1938, he couldn't bear it anymore and he took a trip on his own to visit them. He spent two weeks in Poland with his family, two weeks filled with happiness and love. Could he have imagined as he said goodbye to his father and boarded the train back to Brussels that it would be the last time that he would hug him? The Zionist idea enthralled him, and he'd even considered emigrating to Palestine, but as he had a large family, the fear of not finding work deterred him and he let it slide.

How could he have known that precisely two years later, World War II would break out and his parents and sisters, Sarah and Hannah, would be sent to their cruel death in Auschwitz, and that as a result, his father would never meet his fifth grandchild, Charlie, who was a just a year old? How could he have known that slowly but surely, everything would collapse like a tower of cards because of one crazy man with a ridiculous mustache and a shrill voice and infinite hatred for the Jews? Or that he and his collaborators and the throngs of people supported him?

Could he have imagined, even in his wildest nightmares, that he, his beloved wife and two of his children would be murdered with unparalleled cruelty? Or that they would be among six million other Jews who were part of a satanic and inconceivable plan for the mass extermination of an entire population of people? He looked tenderly at Perla, who, too, had no idea that she had less than four more years to hear her beloved Charlie's wonderful, rolling laughter—not only because she'd be taken to hell and murdered in the Auschwitz concentration camp, but because during the years that followed, until the end of the war, Charlie's laughter would be muted, and suffocating tears, loneliness and terror would take its place.

OCTOBER 1939—OFF TO THE FRENCH ARMY

Eighteen-year-old Israel felt that he had to do something after reading the book *Mein Kampf*, and after the German invasion of Poland in September 1939. On a rather chilly day in October, he woke up about two hours before sunrise and took out the small backpack he had hidden under his bed. He left a short letter in the mailbox that even he found unsatisfactory, and with great excitement, he left home. He off to enlist in the French Army, because as a Polish refugee, he didn't have Belgian citizenship and he couldn't enlist in the Belgian Army.

It was a month after Germany invaded Poland and war broke out between Germany and Britain and France. Although Belgium was still neutral, Israel admired France and he couldn't do nothing when France officially joined the forces fighting against Germany. He did so even though the war was still being called "the phony war" because the guns had not yet thundered, and everyone was waiting to see what would happen next.

The street was empty, the air cold and clear, and his steps echoed in concert with his heartbeat.

Charlie, now two years old, didn't understand where Israel had disappeared to. He used to cover him in kisses and hugs, squeezing bursts of giggles from him when his stubble tickled the soft skin of his face.

Israel was the first to disappear. In the years that followed, Charlie would experience the disappearance of other close and beloved family members, and his developing young mind would build mechanisms of defense and repression to protect it from the pain. These mechanisms would remain so strong and vast, that until his older brother returned to Brussels after the war with medals and stories of heroism, he wouldn't be able to remember that he'd ever existed.

Israel, on the other hand, never forgave himself for leaving so suddenly without so much as a goodbye and abandoning his family without receiving their approval. Only later, as a soldier in the French Army, did he write them a letter explaining and justifying his actions. He couldn't have predicted the trials that his family would have to withstand, or the fate of his parents and siblings. He always felt that maybe if he'd been there, they would have survived, and that feeling grew over the years and became an obsession.

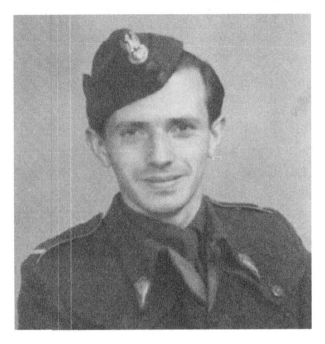

Israel in the army

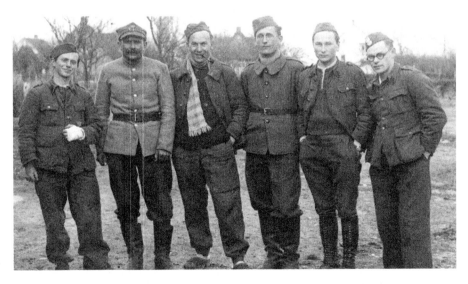

Israel in the prisoner of war camp

MAY 1940—THE FAMILY ESCAPES TO FRANCE

The move from Warsaw to Brussels, which at first seemed like a good idea and was for a few years, couldn't protect the Hilsberg family forever from the more powerful forces of racism and hatred.

Manifestations of anti-Semitism in Germany and Austria, the Nazi Party that was attracting more and more supporters across Europe, and the slowly pervading fear troubled Tola. No one believed any longer that everything would work out fine, and that it was just a passing trend of a few extremists.

One day, Regina returned from school crying bitterly and told them that the teacher, the principal and her friends, were persecuting her because she was Jewish. After Germany declared war on Poland on September 1, 1939, and Israel left, when the thundering cannons drew closer, the family began to think it was time to leave again.

Tola, who had just become engaged to her beloved Adolf, was the main one urging the family to leave, but the first to agree was her mother Perla. Deep down, Perla secretly believed that she would get to see her son Israel again, who was somewhere in France.

And so, when the German invasion of neutral Belgium began, they decided to leave, as did hundreds of thousands of other Belgians, including many non-Jews who remembered the horrors of World War I and the atrocities perpetrated by the Germans in Flanders. It was just before the Germans invaded Brussels that Tola insisted that they act quickly. Her fiancé, Adolph went with the Hilsberg family. They took a few belongings with them, and in the middle of the night they walked fifteen minutes from their home to the nearest train station, Gare Du Midi.

The train was packed to capacity and the family could barely find one seat between them all. Just two hours later, the train stopped because of an air raid that had hit one of the railway cars. All the passengers had to disembark and look for another train. This wasn't the only time they were bombed, and they realized that they could no longer get to Paris, as their train was put out of commission.

So, they had to move on south. They caught another train, which was also switched several times due to the heavy shelling. The trip was long and arduous for everyone. Thousands of refugees packed into the unbearably cramped cars. At times, Moshe made sure that his family held hands so that they wouldn't be separated in the crowd. Perla didn't feel well and nor did Charlie, who clung to his sister Regina. The food ran out, and from time to time, they stopped to freshen up and were helped by kindhearted Red Cross workers, who distributed a little food and drink to the hungry refugees.

After traveling for a few days, the family arrived with a few other Jewish families in the picturesque town of Montegut-Lauragais in the Haute-Garonne region.

The village was six miles from the town of Revel, and they disembarked at the village station because that was where the train stopped. They were a small group among hundreds of Jewish refugees from Belgium who arrived in the region and dispersed to a number of various towns.

MAY-OCTOBER 1940—LIVING IN MONTEGUT-LAURAGAIS

The mayor himself came out to greet them all. Moshe and Perla were stunned when they saw a table piled with delicious food, which the mayor had asked the town residents to prepare in advance. With an expression full of compassion and good will, he told them that the town could happily accommodate five Jewish families. Regina and Charlie began to devour the French bread and fresh croissants baked by the nearby bakery. For a moment, the war was forgotten, they were no longer hungry, and Moshe and Perla's hearts were filled with immense optimism. They praised Tola for insisting on leaving for France, took the few belongings they'd brought with them, and went to the presbytery by the church, where they'd generously been given a place to stay by the parish priest.

The atmosphere there was pleasing. They were given spacious rooms on the top floor, beds with clean cotton covers in every room, and there was a large dining room downstairs, a burning fireplace with a white marble mantel, and a spacious kitchen with ceramic pots for the families that were staying with them to use. These were happy times. They ate well, and even received a refugee allowance from the French authorities. This showed that there were decent and generous French people during World War II.

There was, however, a shadow hanging over them. Perla fell ill and became frail and weak. Charlie was looked after by his responsible twelve-year-old

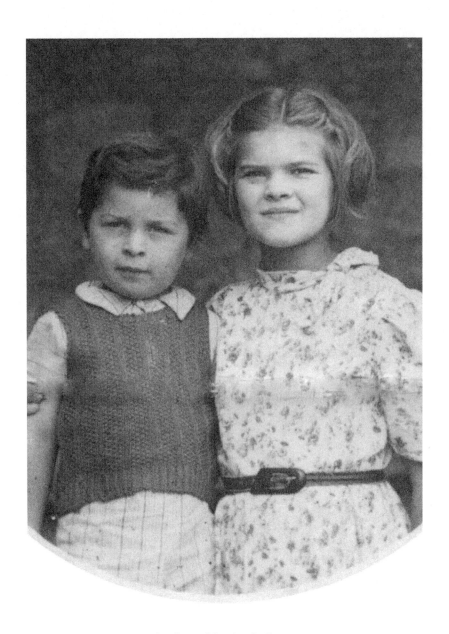

Charlie and Regina in France

sister Regina, who mainly had to keep him away from the deep well next to the presbytery.

They often took walks together, and Regina would take Charlie, now three, to the old and picturesque stone houses, which were far from their home. They would look with interest at the farmland that stretched out to the horizon. Sometimes, they watched the local women washing their clothes in the creek, and on their way back, go past the bakery where the irresistible aroma of baking farm bread filled the air.

On family outings, they usually walked to the delightful neighboring village, Saint Ferréol, which had an artificial lake with a fancy promenade around it. Regina used to go to the local school, where two teachers who taught her took a great liking to her, a mother and her daughter who lived in a small apartment in the school. In the afternoons, she would take Charlie to visit them for tea and homemade cookies. Sometimes she would join a group of children and help the farmers in the area to peel the corn cobs. To make a little money, Tola and her fiancé worked in vineyards near the city of Carcassonne.

The consideration that the locals showed the Jewish refugees reached a new height on Rosh Hashanah, Yom Kippur and Sukkot, when the Jewish families were allowed to turn the church into a synagogue in order to celebrate their holidays. This was certainly an unusual act on the part of the Christians. The statues of the Madonna and the crosses were wrapped and covered in cloth. They found a Jewish butcher in the area, and Moshe Hilsberg even found a shofar. They weren't perturbed by the fact that they didn't have prayer books, since Moshe recreated the prayers, which he wrote on sheets of paper and distributed to the others.

Most importantly—they were together.

SEPTEMBER 2014– RETURN TO REGINA'S "PARADISE"

In the last few years of her life, Regina became more restricted, physically, and she had to use a walker to get about. This made it too difficult for her to visit the area in France where the family lived between May and October 1940. For Regina, that was the happiest time of her youth. She never forgot the village scenery or the surrounding towns, the serene rural atmosphere or the generosity of the people, and she liked to share her memories of those days and talk about them. She urged Shaul to visit the area, take pictures and perhaps talk with the descendants of the people who'd lived there during World War II.

In September of 2014, with the help of his French friends Elizabeth and Philippe Lambert who lived in Provence, Shaul and his wife Dalia visited Montegut-Lauragais, about forty miles from Toulouse, in the Midi Pyrenees region. It was just as Regina had described it—small, well-kept towns scattered in the valleys and on the edges of the hills, creating a lovely, picturesque landscape. Sunflower fields studded the landscape, and the bluish silhouette of the foothills of the Pyrenees glistened on the horizon.

The town church, where the Jewish refugees had celebrated the holidays in the fall of 1940, stood there in all its glory on the hill. Its architecture was typical of the region—an elongated rectangular building alongside an elegant Romanesque style tower. All the statues and paintings of the Madonna and Jesus that the refugees had covered were there. The presbytery was under renovation because it was being converted into a school, but they could go

34

inside to look. Shaul was constantly on the phone with Regina so that they could experience the visit together. Her descriptions turned out to be accurate: the stair railing going up to the second floor was red, the fireplace mantel was white and carved, and the well that their mother was so afraid of stood right by the presbytery, but it was now covered. Later during the visit, Shaul and Dalia met with the mayor and the town representatives at the town hall, including with the son of the mayor back then, and it was profoundly moving. Those who were children or teenagers at the time shared their own memories of that period.

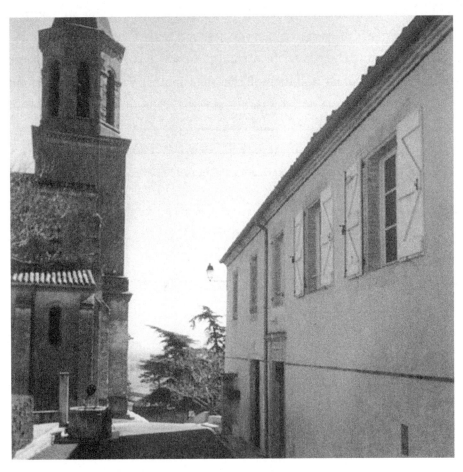

The presbytery, with the well beside it, in 2014

The mayor's wife showed them around, and the tour matched Regina's memories: the local bakery with the smell of bread filling the air...in memory of those days, they bought a huge square of brioche; the promenade along the artificial lake in Saint Ferréol (where the family would take walks on the weekends); the town of Saint Julia, with the main square that resembled a square in Marais in Paris, with the ancient 14th-century market in the center and the antique stores, well known in the area. The tour ended with a rich cassoulet, one of the well-known dishes of the region. During that visit, Dalia and Shaul certainly got to see the nice side of the French.

A week after visiting France, on Rosh Hashanah, Dalia and Shaul went to visit Regina at home in Karkur, spread the photos out for her to look at and told her all about their trip. Regina was thrilled and happy, especially after she got to talk on the phone with the son of the teacher who loved her so. She kept repeating, "I'm so glad that you visited there, it's incredible—I'm getting closure."

It was a Thursday, and they left in the evening. On Saturday, after Rosh Hashanah ended, they talked to her again to see how she was doing. She sounded cheerful and in an uplifted mood. On Sunday, at six o'clock in the morning, the phone rang, startling them. Dalia picked up the receiver, her hand trembling, expecting to hear bad news: it was so early in the morning. And indeed, Pnina, Regina's daughter, told them that she'd just heard from Regina's live-in caregiver that when she came to wake her up to get ready to go to the center for the elderly (where she spent her weekday mornings), she found her dead in her bed. When Shaul and Dalia came to see her in her room, she looked as if she had just fallen asleep, and her face was serene. Although she was already eighty-six years old when she died, her vitality and clarity gave no hint that she would leave this world so quickly. She really had come full circle and she slipped away peacefully.

HELL, OTHERWISE KNOWN AS RIVESALTES

The order from the Vichy government was given in October 1940. The mayor opened the letter delivered by a military envoy and read the order: "You are to immediately gather all the Jews and transfer them to the Rivesaltes internment camp in the South of France." He could not refuse, and with great sorrow, he did as he was told.

The Rivesaltes camp was located on the plain between the Pyrenees and the sea, by the Spanish border, a few miles from Perpignan. The continental climate there was extreme—very cold in the winter and scorching in the summer. It was originally a military camp built in 1938 for housing and training soldiers. On November 12, 1938, following the Spanish Civil War, the French authorities authorized it to be used for confining "unwanted foreigners" such as Spanish refugees. Later it was used as an internment camp for Jews, both during the Vichy regime and following the German invasion of Free France. It was a notorious camp, known as the "Drancy of the free zone" and it reflected badly on France during World War II, who had sole run of it until the Germans took over in November 1942. The deplorable living conditions in the camp, especially for the Jews, were as bad as in the German concentration camps.

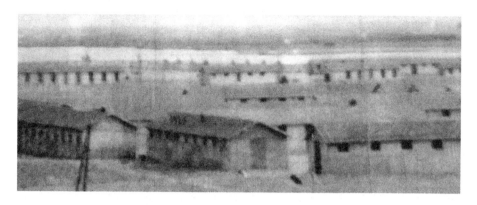

The French concentration camp Rivesaltes

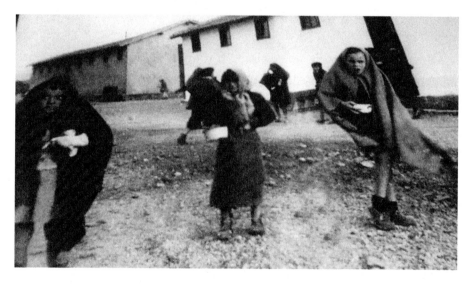

Life in Rivesaltes

The trip to the Rivesaltes internment camp took two days. It was late at night by the time they arrived at gloomy gray camp, the brutal wind was freezing, and they could feel the cold in their bones.

No one welcomed them. They were housed in stuffy long barracks unsuitable even for cattle, about 10-15 feet wide and 200 feet long with only a few windows, some of which were shattered. The roof shingles were broken but they were nonetheless stuffy. They had no mattresses and very few blankets, and so people had to lie on the floor trembling from the cold and moaning weakly from hunger and disease.

Despite the cold, filth and hunger, the gendarmes (French police officers) walked around the camp glaring cruelly at them and barking orders to maintain order and cleanliness. Between the barracks, there were narrow canals and barbed wire fences, but they were forbidden from using the canals as toilets even though the toilets were very far away, too far to walk to during the freezing cold nights.

On the first night, Regina couldn't hold it in anymore and she wet herself. But she wasn't the only one, and they all suffered terribly from the pervasive stench in the closed barracks.

One day, little Charlie was walking through the camp with his mother, and he needed to use the toilet. His mother, realizing that he wouldn't be able to hold it in until they made it to the bathroom, felt for him. After looking carefully around to make sure there were no gendarmes around, she helped him to pull down his trousers by one of the canals. Suddenly, out of nowhere, a gendarme appeared and started to scream at Perla, who became paralyzed with fear. He raised his arm to hit her, but Regina, who had been keeping an eye on Perla and Charlie, remained cool. She quickly ran up to him and grabbed the wing of his coat and said "Please, she doesn't understand French," Regina blurted out to the surprised officer. "I'm sorry. She won't do it again."

The officer changed his mind only after she pleaded with him. Relenting, he walked away muttering curses under his mustache.

They walked around in dirty clothes—they had no laundry facilities, no food, only disease, which was rife. The food rations were meager, and their fear of the unknown kept growing. Every morning, the officers counted them to see if anyone had died or escaped, although it was very difficult to escape since the camp was surrounded by high barbed wire fences and armed police patrolled on motorcycles or walked around the camp with dogs. Moshe and

Marcel worked hard, loading logs onto carts. It was one reason that many later called the camp "the Auschwitz of Southern France."

Still, much to their surprise, a diamond suddenly started to shine in the darkness for Regina.

That diamond was called Mr. Blanc. He was a teacher who organized lessons in French within that hell. He taught them songs and held parties of a sort when they would sing the songs and even dance to them. They performed for the French officers, who were delighted for the cultural respite. Regina cherished those precious hours, which gave her an escape from the hardships and hunger, while Charlie clung constantly to her because Perla was so ill. He was barely three years old and still didn't understand the meaning behind the constant exhausting upheavals.

Perla grew even weaker, but so did all of them. They became sick and were covered in lice that made them itchy all over.

Then, the Hilsberg family heard awful rumors regarding their future. Although Belgium was occupied by the Germans on May 10, 1940, the situation of the Belgian Jews was still tolerable, certainly in comparison to their own situation in France. Tola, the living and driving force of the family, was the first to understand this. "We have to run away again," she said. "We can't get to Spain because the Pyrenees are too high and steep, and we don't have money to hire a guide to take us across the border. Mama doesn't feel well and won't be able to withstand the journey and that leaves us no choice but to return to Belgium," she explained to everyone.

It never entered her mind to abandon her family and escape with her fiancé to Spain. After all, the two youngsters could have fled for their lives across the mountains. No, Tola was loyal to her family and she wouldn't hear of such an option. Instead, she organized their escape from the camp.

Somehow, perhaps because of her beauty and charm (Regina claimed it was because she gave away a precious stone that she had kept), she managed to bribe a gendarme, and one night in March 1941, they escaped from the camp and set out for Montpellier. It was probably well into the winter of 1941, because the weather remained cold the entire way, and it was still winter when they arrived in Brussels.

MARCH 1941—FLEEING BACK TO BRUSSELS

What made the Hilsberg family return to the place from which they'd fled? What made those hundreds of thousands of Jews throughout Europe stay, even after they had the opportunity to escape? Twenty-twenty hindsight is easy, but if it had been the right move, their optimism and courage would have been admired. In retrospect it is easy to judge the situation and say, "Oh, they were complacent, too naïve."

One cannot judge, however, especially not the Hilsberg family. What choice did they have, with Perla so ill and weak? The option of leaving for Spain and going on that difficult trek was never an option. And it is important to remember that at the beginning of 1941, the horrific orders and instructions issued in Germany, Eastern Europe and now in occupied Vichy France, had not yet been given in Belgium.

Word of the Final Solution to the Jewish Question and the plan to exterminate the Jews had not yet reached the Hilsberg family. Although the situation of the Belgian Jews wasn't good, it was still better than in neighboring countries. There is no doubt that if they'd stayed at Rivesaltes, the whole family would have been wiped out, because eventually everyone from the camp was transported to the Drancy camp and from there to Auschwitz. This is what happened under the French government in Vichy to all the captives in camps across the South of France. Charlie and Regina would have been sent to the gas chambers or died of starvation, abuse or disease beforehand. At least the escape that Tola arranged saved Regina and Charlie and granted the family another year together. Although life was difficult and tenuous, it was also full of warmth and love.

In June 2012, Dalia and Shaul visited the Rivesaltes camp near Perpignan with their friends Philippe Lambert, and Jacqueline and David Inowlocki. If not for the monuments to the gypsies and the Jews that now stand at the entrance to the camp, it would have felt like they'd traveled back in time. The long barracks in the neglected expanses of nettles and thorns remained as if the refugees had just been there. The windows were shattered, the doors broken, and the neglect was as rampant as it had been back then. There were fields of crops around the camp, which must have been there at the beginning of the war, making the visitors wonder why the prisoners had suffered so severely from such severe starvation that killed hundreds of them, as they got no help from the French. On their visit, they were told by the local guide that there had been plans to demolish the camp and build a real estate project in its place. Only the protest of Holocaust survivors, led by former French Minister of Health Ms. Simone Veil, prevented the plan from being implemented, and instead a memorial museum was established in the abandoned camp.

The historical documents relating to the camp and the view of the sleep slopes of the Pyrenees fully convinced Dalia and Shaul that without money and papers, the family really had no choice but to return to Brussels.

The journey home took about a month. With the help of the French underground, they caught a ride on a truck and arrived in Montpellier, where they shared a single room between the seven of them at a shabby and filthy hotel. They were still itchy from the lice and had to listen anxiously to little Charlie coughing terribly after he caught whooping cough. Still, at least they were given a change of clothes, and at least they now had hope again. They didn't have papers or documents, but they were lucky enough not to run into the Germans on their way to Beziers, only the French. From there, they continued to Paris and again, stayed at a tiny, musty hotel on Rue du Temple. They then found a roundabout way back to Brussels.

All that they went through along the way was immediately forgotten when they walked back into their dear apartment in Brussels and found it just as they'd left it. They reached an agreement with the landlord, and for a few weeks, they felt as if they had returned to heaven.

Their happiness reached a peak at the wedding. About two weeks after returning home, Tola married her beloved Adolph. In a modest ceremony in the synagogue, in front of a few guests and before curfew began, they swore to each other that they would never part, and did not imagine how quickly they would have to put their vows to the test. Tola and Adolph moved into a small street in the Saint-Gilles district, not far from Tola's parents.

THE FIRST SIGNS OF DEATH—THE YELLOW BADGE

Sometimes death comes slowly and nests in the body for months. The yellow badge that the Jews of Brussels were ordered to wear in June 1942 appeared suddenly, like the first signs of melanoma on the skin: the person still feels healthy inside, but the cancer is slowly spreading to all the organs of their body.

And then more signs appeared: Jewish children were forbidden to attend schools with non-Jewish children; Jews were banned from trade and other professions, aside from providing medical care to other Jews; Jews were prohibited from living outside certain cities; and they were also prohibited from leaving the country. A curfew between 6:00 PM and 6:00 AM was imposed, and if that wasn't enough, in November 1941, the Nazi regime created the Belgian Judenrat AJB (Association des Juifs de Belgique), a buffer between the Belgian authorities and the Jews that included only Jews with Belgian citizenship. This meant that it represented only 10 percent of Belgian Jewry. In time, the AJB was harshly criticized as many believed that they cooperated more than necessary with the German authorities. The Nazis demanded that the AJB provide detailed lists of Jews with their accurate addresses, including apartment numbers and floors. The Jewish underground tried to destroy the lists but failed. Sixty years later, Shaul found the document recording the entire Hilsberg family, including himself at two-and-a-half years old, in the archives of the Jewish Holocaust Museum in Mechelen.

But the fear of death shrinks when it encounters love. And Tola was in love and enjoying her new marriage, even under the difficult conditions.

At first, Perla continued to go out to the street to meet up with Tola, find out how she and Adolph were managing and to give her a little of their food, which was in short supply. But the mysterious illness had made her weak and Regina braved the Nazi-infested streets instead. She would give Tola coal and food and find the supplies that Perla asked for. Regina had an Aryan appearance and was extraordinarily resourceful. Bravely, she would remove the yellow badge and walk down the street, her step relaxed as she smuggled the goods passed the stern officers, trying to disguise her nervousness and racing heart.

MARCEL

August 1942 was a hot month. Marcel, a good-looking boy with blazing, kind eyes, frowned and repeated, "I've made up my mind and that's that."

Perla started crying and Moshe bit his lip. "It's a trap," Moshe tried again. "Please don't go."

Marcel shook his head, feeling sorry for his father for being so suspicious. "They said that it's a labor camp, not a concentration camp, do you understand?" He spoke softly, trying to convince Moshe that there was no need for concern.

Perla picked up the recruitment order, but she couldn't read it through the tears.

"The AJB assured me," Marcel argued, "that no harm would come to you if I enlisted to go to this labor camp, so what's the problem? I'm young, I'm strong, I'll work a little and then I'll come back to you."

After a tense silence, Moshe stated with determination, "Under no circumstances. I won't allow it."

Marcel didn't argue. He knew full well that it was pointless. He sighed as if he'd accepted the decision and went to his room. The next morning, on August 4, he wrote a short farewell letter to his parents and left home, never to return.

He was the second to disappear from Charlie's life.

Marcel paid for his naivete with his life. He was put on the first transport to Auschwitz along with another 998 youths who believed that they were saving their families by enlisting to go to the labor camp.

The German extermination machine had now begun to wipe out the Jews of Belgium as well, and the youth were at the top of the list, perhaps because the Germans wanted first and foremost to get rid of any possible resistance from the young, as they did in Slovakia.

As soon as they arrived at the camp, 254 youths were murdered. Only a few from that transport survived until the end of the war.

In the morning, when Moshe and Perla realized that Marcel was gone, they ran to the train station where they found a note that Marcel had thrown out for them. The note indicated that he'd realized he'd fallen into a trap.

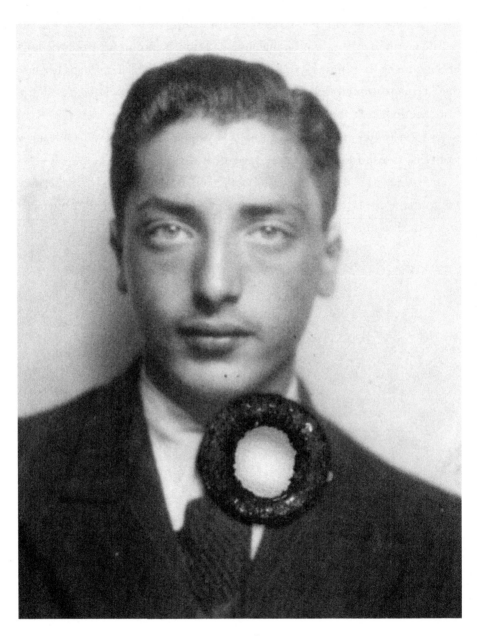

Marcel

TOLA

If the yellow badge symbolized a melanoma blemish, then the opening of Caserne Dossin heralded the spread of malignant metastases to the internal organs. Caserne Dossin (Dossin Barracks formerly belonged to the Belgian army and was located in the city of Mechelen, between Antwerp and Brussels). Trains carrying 26 transports were sent directly from the Caserne Dossin after tracks were laid right to the entrance. All in all, 26,000 Jews were on those trains, including 5,400 children—about 43% of pre-war Belgium's 60,000 Jews. The hunts and raids on the streets became more frequent, and every day, more and more Jews disappeared from their homes.

Regina bravely and willingly met Tola every day, as Perla asked her to. One day, Regina was waiting for Tola at their usual spot, but Tola didn't show up. Instead, Regina saw a convoy of German soldiers crossing the street.

Regina quickly crossed to the other side and hurried to Tola's apartment. One of the neighbors told her the bitter news: there had been a major raid the night before, and all the Jews from Rue de Merode were led away by the Germans. Regina ran home in tears. Before going inside, she stopped to wipe away the tears, wondering how she would tell her mother.

Perla understood for herself. The look in Regina's eyes was so hard and so sad that Perla merely asked, "How did it happen?"

"There was a raid," Regina replied in a voice that sounded like a stranger's voice.

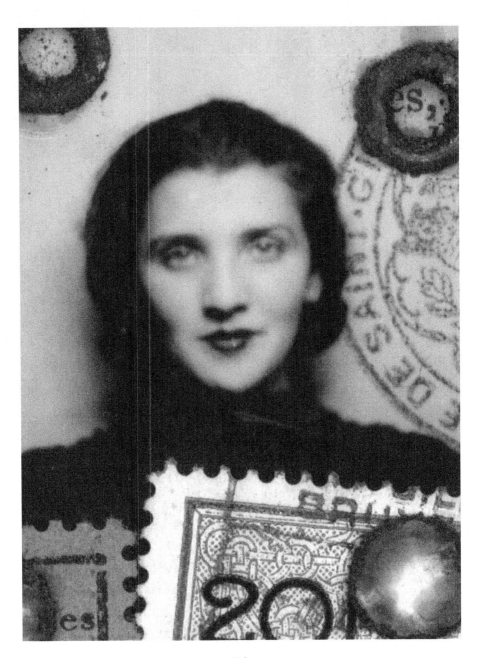

Tola

Perla went to the window, looked down at the horizon and said, as if to herself, "They took my sunshine away, my Tola."

Two days later, in September 1942, beautiful 22-year-old Tola and her new husband Adolph sat huddled and trembling on Transport No. 9 to Auschwitz. He squeezed her hand and she looked deep into his eyes. They were very young, and brave, but in that moment, they felt hopeless. The train lugged them away from Brussels, parting them not only from their past but also from their future. They would no longer sleep in each other's arms under the blankets, they would not have children, they would not have interesting careers or hobbies. They would freeze in the cold, they would starve, and then be taken naked and humiliated to the gas chambers. They would not even have their own graves.

And they would suffer these punishments because of their unforgivable sin of being born Jewish.

Tola was the third to disappear from Charlie's life.

Over the next few weeks, the family, which had shrunk to just the parents, Regina and Charlie, would barely survive. Moshe was taken with his sewing machine to work for the Germans in a sweatshop and was away from home from dawn to dusk. He felt that his life was running out, and it was difficult for him to cheer up his sick wife and make his two remaining children happy. Food was scarce and they quickly sold off their household belongings to buy more.

BRUSSELS—BEHIND A THIN WALL

It was in late 1942 or early 1943. Thirteen-year-old Regina sat tremoring in her room. The shrill, menacing voice of Adolf Hitler bursting from the neighbors' radio resounded in her ears and in her tender soul. There was no need to understand the language in order to detect the hatred and madness. Fear flowed in her arteries and she cringed on her bed as if his words were poisoned arrows shot personally at her. She was not an adult, but she was already mature enough to understand a thing or two about this world. She got out of bed, smoothed a stray strand of her long hair from her forehead, left the apartment, skipped down the stairs, waved to the concierge, checked again that she'd remembered to take the shoes that needed the skilled hands of the cobbler, and opened the gate.

She looked down the street and froze.

The street was barricaded, and the Gestapo were loading terrified Jews into trucks. "It's a raid," she whispered to herself as she watched a group of soldiers in SS uniforms marching towards her home.

Her heart, which had stopped for a moment, was now beating wildly. Her mind was as active as a battlefield and her reaction was sharp and immediate. She took a step back, closed the gate, passed by the astonished concierge who crossed herself, and flew up the stairs back to their apartment. It was the fastest and longest climb in her life. Trying to catch her breath, she told her parents: "The Germans are here. We have to run away."

Her mother, who was setting the table for Friday dinner, turned very pale, and the dish she was holding dropped from her hand. She looked at Charlie playing on the carpet in the living room. She picked him up in her arms and turned toward the door. Moshe started to look for the key to his tie room in the attic on the sixth floor.

"Quick!" Regina cried. "We don't have time! Let's go!"

Cold sweat appeared on Moshe's forehead. "I can't find the key," he muttered, and Perla interrupted him, "It doesn't matter, Moshe, let's go up. Now."

Moshe locked the apartment door so that the Germans would think the family had left and they began to climb the many stairs to the attic. They could hear that the Nazi soldiers were downstairs. As they sped up the stairs, their Belgian neighbor opened his door and looked at them in astonishment. Regina held her finger to her lips, signaling him to be quiet. He nodded and closed the door. Seconds later, the family was standing in the attic looking for a place to hide. The tie room, where Moshe kept his stock and was hoping to hide, was locked.

They had no choice but to hide behind the wall in the center of the attic, which was open on both sides. Both parents, Regina, and five-year-old Charlie stood behind the wall, trying to silence their pounding hearts. They could hear terrible shouting from below. The Nazis had burst into the butcher's apartment on the first floor. His wife was in an advanced stage of pregnancy and her screams were etched permanently in Charlie's heart. To this day, he can still hear them.

"Don't take him, please!" she begged. But the uniformed men ignored her pleas, and the butcher was dragged away like some meaningless object. Perla took a step toward the stairs. She had to save the butcher's pregnant wife, but Regina grasped her hand firmly and whispered to her, "Stop! We're all going to die."

Perla kept muttering the Shema prayer, "Hear O Israel, the Lord our God, the Lord is One." Moshe's heart contracted in pain. He felt terribly guilty because he couldn't find the key to the tie room and felt the custom-made ties tightening around his neck.

They could hear the sound of hobnailed jackboots approaching their hiding place in the attic. They held their breath. Charlie's eyes widened in terror. Someone, maybe it was his father, pushed a rag he found into his mouth and warned him not to take it out. They all leaned tremoring against the wall and holding each other's hands. Moshe moved his lips silently in prayer.

A soldier came into the attic but tired from the steep climb, he leaned against the wall and lit a cigarette. On the other side of the wall, just a few inches away, three of the four of them were certain that those were their last moments. In a minute, after smoking his cigarette, the soldier would turn and take just two steps to his right or left and see them hiding.

Five-year-old Charlie didn't think about death. The concept was still too abstract for him to understand its meaning. He did, however, feel terrified in every inch of his soul. He looked at his parents, who at the last minute would always manage to save him from danger. He trusted them as devoutly as one who believes in God, and now, for the first time in his life, he could feel their vulnerability…and something inside him broke.

"Anymore dirty Jews there?" The soldier's commander shouted to him from below, the harsh German sounding to Charlie like heavy boots on gravel. The soldier took one last puff of his cigarette, calmly blew smoke rings and threw the cigarette on the floor, then ground it with his heel to put it out.

He was still tired from climbing the stairs and he was too lazy to walk around the attic.

"Nix!" he shouted to his commander. "Nothing here."

They all breathed a sigh of relief but stayed in the attic until evening just to be safe. The rag had already been taken out of Charlie's mouth, but he didn't cry, and he didn't shout. He said nothing.

Many years would pass before he agreed to talk about that night. For many years, he would keep it in and avoid not only speaking of it but even remembering. Whenever there was imminent danger in his life, he stifled his feelings and look at death with astonishing restraint. He made the choice to have an imaginary rag stuffed in his mouth.

Even then, his young and courageous soul had the wonderful survival instinct that told him to bury and forget that moment and all the other horrible moments yet to come if he wanted to continue living. Not forever, but until he was strong enough to deal with the wounds; until he had lived enough life, and had enough laughter, love and professional success. Until he could bravely overcome his fears and felt that not only did he no longer need to silence his inner self, but that it was time to connect all of his parts and share his story, not only for his soul to heal but also for the sake of his children, grandchildren and any child who is suffering. And also so that they would not lose hope and to help them to remember that a person can experience unimaginably complex and scarring childhood traumas and still come out of the darkness and shadows and find light and hope...and achieve everything that they dream of achieving.

Regina and Charlie spent that night at the concierge, Madame Lacroix, and the following days and nights with their next-door neighbor, Madame Claes, all the while watching their apartment to see if anyone came and went and if their parents were at home. Then, for a few weeks, they moved around from place to place with their parents, sometimes sleeping over, including with Hungarian acquaintances of theirs. They were afraid to go home.

Regina would go out every few days to their apartment to fetch groceries and fabric to sell, mainly to buy coal to keep warm, as the winter was harsh. Naturally, she would leave her yellow badge behind. She would rip it off her clothes, and thanks to her Aryan features, she could walk around without being stopped. It's hard to believe that a girl, barely fourteen-and-a-half years old, was actually the mainstay of the family. The concierge's son would open the door for her and help her, and she would go down to the dark basement with a flashlight in her hand and carry sacks of coal and groceries on her back in the dark and cold. She sold her father's remaining fabric to a neighbor.

One day she returned to the Hungarian family's apartment and found people there in Nazi uniform. These were Belgians who had disguised themselves as Nazis in order to rob people. Moshe had jumped over the porch to escape. Regina burst into tears and one of the neighbors invited her in. Later, with the help of their friend Mr. Kremer, the one who convinced them to emigrate to Belgium, they found an abandoned apartment and stayed there for a while.

Regina could sense Charlie's constant fear. He would curl up in her lap and in Perla's lap whenever he heard a car on the street and ask, "Mama, are the Germans coming?"

They eventually started running out of places to hide and were left with no choice but to return to their apartment. Perla fell ill again, and Regina took her by tram to the school that had been converted into a hospital. The manager said that he wasn't allowed to accept Jews, but nonetheless he agreed to hospitalize her. It was hard for Regina to visit her. One day the manager informed Regina that she had to take her mother away, otherwise the whole hospital would be in jeopardy. Having no choice, Regina took Perla home.

After all those difficulties, Moshe and Perla realized with a heavy heart that they had no choice; that in order to save the children, they had to hand them over to the Jewish underground, the CDJ (Committee de Defence des Juifs). At least they would stand a chance of surviving.

The Jewish underground movement, the CDJ, was established in 1942 by eight people to create a counterweight to the AJB, who cooperated with the Germans. Together with the Belgian underground, they aimed to protect the Jewish population.

THE COMMITTEE FOR THE PROTECTION OF JEWS (COMMITTEE DE DEFENCE DES JUIFS)

First and foremost, the Germans wanted to exterminate the Jewish children.

Aside from their satanic plan to destroy the entire Jewish people, whoever and wherever they were, they were also concerned that when the children grew up, they would want to avenge the murder of their parents and grandparents. As such, they planned with evil cunning to carry out their plan without the world finding out. Their obsessive persecution of the Jewish children remains incomprehensible and unbearable to this day. Even when they were facing a crushing defeat, they did not give up but continued to pursue them to the end. An estimated 1.5 million Jewish children were murdered during the Holocaust. In fact, the sign at the Jewish Museum in Mechelen states that no Jewish child under the age of 13 sent from Mechelen to Auschwitz came back alive.

It is worth noting that a significant part of the Belgian people—from members of the royal family, the Catholic clergy, the governmental and municipal staff and activists from various institutions and organizations to blue-collar workers and peasants—behaved morally and admirably and did not succumb to fear. Dowager Queen Elisabeth of Belgium (who was also awarded the title of Righteous Among the Nations) played an important role in the rescue operation, and although the religious establishment did not issue a formal statement regarding its opposition to expulsion, Catholic institutions, and especially the simple clergy, agreed to hide Jewish children in convents, orphanages, convalescence homes, and more. About 55 percent of Belgian Jews survived, a much higher percentage than that of its neighbor, the Netherlands. After the war, many wondered why more Belgian than Dutch Jews were saved. One explanation for this was the military rule in Belgium, which the Germans defined as Roman, whereas they defined the Netherlands as Germanic. The military rulers were concerned mainly with military security and economic exploitation of the occupied state and did not see the extermination of the Jews as their primary mission. Still, in the summer of 1942, following political pressure, the picture changed, surprising the Jewish community with the AJB's recruitment of young people to labor camps, a ruse that turned out to be nothing but the first transport of Jews to Auschwitz.

Then, in the following months and at a dizzying pace, a third of the Jews who perished in the Holocaust were sent to their deaths. Still, both the Jewish and the Belgian populations soon responded and came up with rescue operations involving all the layers of society. Undoubtedly, the Belgians acted according to their conscience and feelings far more than their neighbors did, but perhaps this was also due to the impact of the traumatic atrocities committed by the Germans in their country during World War I. The extremely active Communist Party, which played an important part in the resistance movements of both the foreign Jewish refugees and of the general population, also contributed to this. One of the important goals of the CDJ was to save Jewish children, after clearly recognizing that if the adults couldn't be saved, it was vital to save the children (whose fate to be sent to the gas chambers had been determined).

This required comprehensive and meticulous planning. The man responsible for the children's rescue operation on behalf of the Jewish underground was Maurice Heiber, who was also a member of the AJB, the Judenrat, which gave him a cover for his underground activities. The underground also cooperated with ONE, the Belgian National Agency for Children, run by Yvonne

Nevejean (who was bestowed the title of Righteous Among the Nations). It should be noted that although there was organized activity around Brussels initiated by two women, Werber and Perelman, which led to the hiding of over 300 children, there is no doubt that the CDJ's contribution was cardinal.

Gradually, word spread through the Jewish community that children could be saved by contacting the Jewish underground through agents who had infiltrated the ranks of the various organizations such as ONE, the Red Cross and official Jewish organizations. There was also a rumor concerning secret mailboxes that had been placed in a number of places.

EVERY CHILD HAS A NAME AND A SECRET CODE

Organizing the challenging operation of saving Jewish children required a number of complex and difficult actions. These included making a list of children to hide and finding places to hide them. Some were hidden with Christian Belgian families, usually simple, hardworking families who would be willing to hide a child or two. Others were hidden in convents, churches, boarding schools, and on farms and in castles. They had to issue forged identity cards bearing non-Jewish names and baptismal certificates and obtained food stamps, because without them, there was no way to ensure that the hidden children would have anything to eat. The children also had to look like the people hiding them. After all, a child with black hair in a family of blonds would have attracted attention.

On top of that, they had to ensure the security of these children with monetary compensation. They used donations from wealthy private sources, the Joint (American Jewish Joint Distribution Committee - is the largest Jewish humanitarian organization in the world) and the Belgian government in exile in Britain for funding. Funds were transferred by couriers who risked their lives, or they were parachuted in.

Finally, a very sophisticated system of codes was created to record the children's whereabouts, identities and real names so that they could be located. The complex records were kept by members of the underground (according to Andree Geulen, Yvonne Jospa and Esther Heiber) who divided the codes between them: one list contained the children's real names and a numerical code; a second list contained the parents' names and addresses with the secret code; the third included the children's fake names along with the same code; a fourth listed the children's fake names and their real dates of birth, without specifying the place of birth, as well as the name of the person hiding them, but without the address or code of the place where the child was hidden; and the last list contained the names of the institutions or families hiding the children, along with the secret code and the institution code. The codebooks were divided between them and hidden in a number of places. While some of the brave volunteers were caught by the Germans and sent to prison, the lists never fell into their hands.

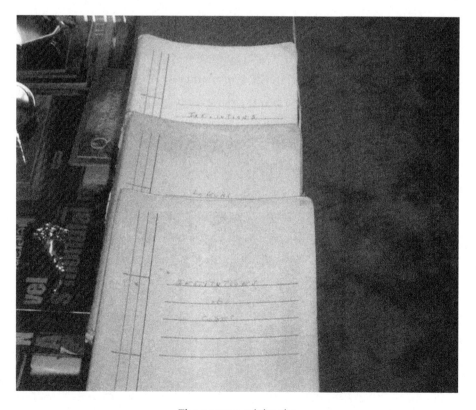

The secret codebooks

A great deal of effort was put into creating the organizational structure and selecting a team suitable for field work. This team included 12 women, some of whom were Jewish social workers, such as Yvonne Jospa, Esther Heiber and Ida Sterno, who obtained fake documents to help them move around and do their jobs. Others, such as Andree Geulen and Brigitte Moons, who weren't Jewish, also volunteered for the mission.

Children over the age of seven or eight were handed over to general Belgian institutions that cooperated willingly, while the younger children were sent to families, usually working-class. The men of the families were often tram drivers or blue-collar workers.

After the war, one of the "angels" involved in rescuing the children testified: "We didn't give the parents their children's addresses because we were afraid that they would visit them and put them in danger. The children were considered Belgian for all intents and purposes and spoke fluent French, whereas their p0arents usually spoke Yiddish or broken French, which could pose quite a threat to both themselves and to the person hiding their child."

Regular visits to the hidden children were necessary to make sure they were being treated well by the families and to determine the level of danger they were in from the Nazis.

This was determined also by tips they would get, sometimes from postal workers. They would often (and very carefully) open official orders sent by mail and leak plans for raids and arrests to the underground.

Sometimes there were misunderstandings between the children and the families hiding them, and someone from the Jewish underground, who kept a constant eye on the children and on their temporary homes, would have to solve any issues.

For instance, Maurice Heiber testified, he said that one day he was called by a Belgian family to take away the Jewish child they were hiding because he'd stolen the baby Jesus doll from their child. They said that they weren't willing to risk themselves for a thieving child.

Sternly, Heiber scolded him: "These people have been so good to you, why did you repay them by stealing the baby Jesus doll from them? You've made them very sad."

In tears, the boy replied, "Not at all, I didn't steal the baby Jesus doll, I only hid it!"

Heiber asked, "Why did you hide it? What happened?"

The boy responded, "They told me that Jesus was born Jewish, and I was afraid that the Germans would take him away, as they might take me."

When the family heard the story, their eyes filled with tears and they agreed to let the child stay.

Hospitals and sanatoriums that would hide Jewish children temporarily before they were sent to permanent hiding places would come up with methods to protect the children. At one sanatorium, the medical staff applied a contrasting material to the children's skin before x-raying them to fabricate images of lungs with tuberculosis damage. The Germans, afraid of dying from the infectious disease, kept their distance.

THERE WERE MANY RIGHTEOUS—BUT ONLY ONE ANDREE GEULEN

Five-year-old Charlie's personal beam of light was called Andree Geulen. She was born in 1921, and despite her bourgeois and affluent origins, she was a rebellious girl, a black sheep whose actions were frowned upon by her parents and her family. Even before World War II broke out, the girl with an extraordinary personality decided to take a stand and do all that she could to help the civil war refugees fleeing from Spain and Franco's fascist reign of terror. She helped to organize food and accommodations for them.

Andree Geulen was a beautiful blonde Belgian with blue eyes, and no man could remain indifferent to her radiant feminine presence when she passed by the street. She was only 21 years old when she decided to join the underground.

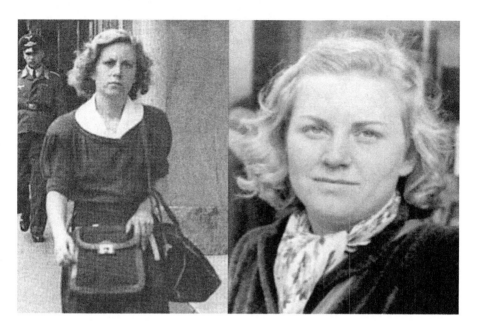

Andree Geulen

It all began by chance. She was working as a boarding school counselor, and one night, when she hugged one of the little children, he brushed her hair aside and whispered in her ear that his name was Simon, not Rene. She looked at him in surprise and then he went on to tell her that he was Jewish, and that's why they gave him another name—so that the Germans wouldn't catch him. That was how she learned for the first time about the hidden Jewish children being saved from the concentration camps to which their parents were sent.

A few days later, in the dead of night, they heard heavy, insistent knocking at the door. Five Gestapo officers entered the boarding school. The children stood to the right side of the classroom and looked wide-eyed at the violent Nazis, who told the Jewish children to move to the left and all the non-Jewish children to stay on the right. The Jewish children, who knew well what confessing to being Jewish meant, were terrified and stayed where they were, on the right. One of the officers was tall and thin with a mustache like Hitler's.

Suddenly, like a bad magician, he pulled out a frightening whip and thundered threateningly at the children. "Any child I catch lying," he declared, narrowing his eyes, "will receive a terrible whipping from me that he'll remember until the day he dies." Then he turned to Andree, who was in shock, and berated her, "How are you not ashamed, a blonde, blue-eyed Aryan such as yourself, teaching little Jewish fleas and looking after them? They must be crushed while they're still small."

Andree recovered quickly, put on her best and most beautiful poker face and replied calmly, "There are no Jewish children here, Mr. Officer, and in any case, how exactly am I meant to tell the difference between a Jewish and a non-Jewish child?" Then, in a bold move that could have cost her imprisonment, she added a bitter, mocking comment: "And how can it be, esteemed gentlemen, that you, the descendants of the glorious Schiller and Goethe, are declaring war on innocent children?"

No one said a word and the officer in charge stared into her shining blue eyes and slowly succumbed to her feminine charm. He muttered something about having other jobs to take care of and told his subordinates to follow him. Pale and breathless, Andree could finally breathe a sigh of relief and sit down to hide her trembling knees from the children.

On another occasion, she learned that during one of the school vacations, the Germans had raided a boarding school and arrested Jewish children who had stayed there instead of going home. On the day they returned from vacation, when the other Jewish children were about to enter the school, Geulen stood courageously at the gate, preventing them from going in, basically saving their lives.

Due to these events, Ida Sterno, one of the leaders of CDJ rescue team, needed women like Andree Geulen and she asked her to join the rescue operations. Andree naturally and willingly agreed. She felt very attached to the Jewish children, and she found the thought of them being hurt so outrageous that she decided to become more involved. Risking her own life, she volunteered to take on a more active role in the Belgian underground's efforts to hide the children.

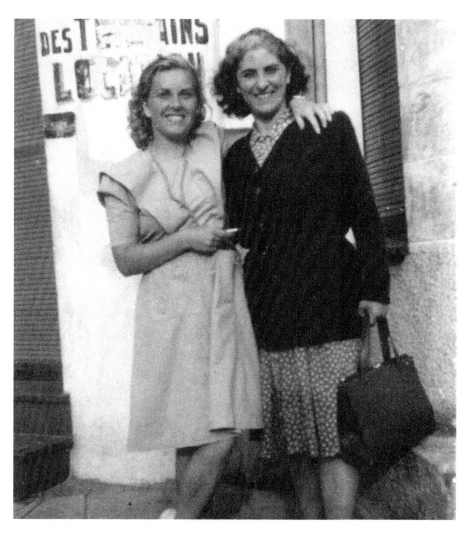

Andree Geulen and Ida Sterno During the War

Ida Sterno was responsible for finding suitable hiding places for the children, and she kept her eye on the young, beautiful and energetic girl Andree, who put her heart and soul into the project. She assigned her the most dangerous and significant job of taking the children from their parents to their hiding places. This involved physical danger, but above all, mental trauma, for she was to witness the most chilling moments of separation imaginable: between parents and their children. Sterno's keen instincts told her to choose a woman who would inspire confidence from all parties; a woman who would be trusted by mothers who had to hand over their precious children to her; one who the Nazi soldiers would trust and who because of her Aryan looks, wouldn't arrest her, even when she was seen walking along with a suspicious-looking group of children; and a woman who radiated beauty and serenity, even when terrified and tense.

Andree Geulen certainly met all of her requirements, and Ida Sterno soon saw that her instincts hadn't deceived her.

Slowly, and despite the difficulties, especially the emotional one of taking the children from their parents, young Andree gained experience and learned from her colleagues' failures. She learned how to talk to distraught parents, how to make an immediate connection with the children, especially the little ones who did not always understand where they were being taken. She learned to smile falsely at SS or Wehrmacht soldiers when they noticed she had a child with her who was not her own. She would notice them trying to work out how such a young lady (who looked even younger than her twenty years) could have a six-year-old child, for example, or even several children.

After the war, Andree said that the hardest part of it all was taking the children from their parents. More than once she witnessed scenes that tore her heart to shreds. The older children would console the parents and the younger ones would cling to her in despair. The children fell in love with her, and the parents fully trusted her. Later, she admitted that if she'd had children of her own at the time, she doubted that she would have managed to carry out the mission.

A brave and defiant person, her rescue operations were at times spontaneous and bold. She once arrived at the home of a family, a father with six children, who had just received an order to report immediately with his children, along with the other Jews. Without hesitation, Andree tore the order to pieces and led the father and his six children to a hiding place. Thanks to her, the whole family survived.

One of her jobs was to acquire food stamps, which were so essential for the children. When she went one morning to the food stamp office, one of the clerks began to ask her bothersome questions: Why did she need so many stamps"? Who exactly did she work for?... and so on. A police officer who was watching asked her to leave immediately so she wouldn't get into trouble with the Gestapo and assured her that if she came back the next day, he would help her to get stamps. All night she thought about his suggestion, afraid that it was just a trap. Still, when morning came, she took the risk and went directly to the food stamp office. The officer kept his promise, thus ensuring a supply of food for the children for another while longer.

Andree would take the children to their allocated hiding places by train, on bicycles, carts of hay and on foot. Luckily, she was never arrested, even though she was close to it a number of times.

She lived with Ida Sterno in an apartment where they hid some of the codebooks under the tiles. At one point, Ida Sterno was caught by the Gestapo and taken to their interrogation center, where she was severely tortured (which later affected her life expectancy). The underground had no idea to what extent she could withstand torture. They were very afraid that the codebooks would be found, which would have allowed the Germans to locate the thousands of hidden children. Andree and another member of the underground put their lives on the line, and in the dead of night, climbed through the window into their apartment and removed the codebooks from under the flooring.

The Germans never did get their hands on any of the codebooks, and the lives of some 3,000 Jewish Belgian children were saved thanks to the CDJ and the 12 brave women of the rescue team, including Andree Geulen.

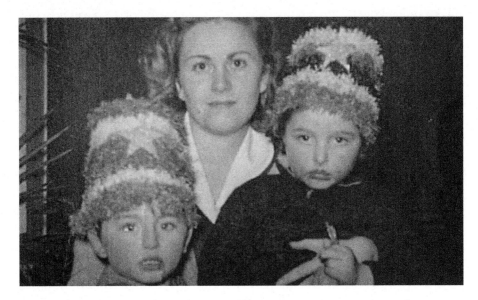

Andree Geulen with children during a rescue mission

After the war, while completing her degree in social work, Andree Geulen continued working to help Jewish children find their families. She met a Jewish law student at university, married him and raised a wonderful family. She stayed in close contact with the Jewish community and enjoyed nothing more than hearing jokes in Yiddish.

In 1989, this wonderful woman was awarded the title of Righteous Among the Nations.

In 2007, when Shaul Harel organized an international conference of the hidden Jewish Belgian children, she was awarded honorary citizenship of Israel in a solemn ceremony held at Yad Vashem.

MAMA, DON'T CRY
(OR THE JUDGEMENT OF SOLOMON)

She knew she had to let go but she just couldn't release her grip. Her hands felt glued to his skin. Because although she understood and had even initiated sending her remaining two children away to be hidden, when the moment of truth came, she became terrified, and an icy feeling filled her heart. So she clung to him, to her sweet, little boy, who despite her tremors and distress, never cried or caused any fuss. He only filled her heart with happiness with his smiling face and rolling laughter. She held him so close to her warm heart that she almost suffocated him, but he didn't complain. No one complains when they feel loved, even if they are hugged too tight, even if they are squeezed. He had no idea why his mother was hugging him like that and crying at the same time; why she loved him so but was sad, too. Where did she suddenly find such strength in her hands? Most of the time she lay weak and pale in bed, and Regina told him that Mama was ill and was not to be disturbed. Where had that sudden burst of energy come from?

He noticed that his sister Regina was also very upset, and was muttering "Mama, don't cry," (his father, as usual was at the sweatshop). He also didn't understand who that beautiful woman was, holding her arms out to him, and why his mother was handing him to her. Although the beautiful woman promised that she would take him to a village where he would take care of cute little farm animals, for some reason he wasn't happy. Nor did he cry because he didn't understand. He never imagined that it would be the last time he would ever see his mother or feel her arms envelop him so protectively and tenderly. Years later, he would say that he couldn't remember that moment—and he really couldn't. It is only in telenovelas that goodbye scenes are so long and dramatic. There were no violins playing when Charlie Hilsberg was passed from his mother's arms into the arms of the stranger, and the only person crying was Perla, who bit her lip as she made the most painful concession she had ever had to make in her life: she gave up the child she so loved, so that he would live. Never had the story of the judgement of Solomon been so fitting to a situation than this one…the mothers were as heroic as the Jewish heroes of the revolt and of the underground. They gave their children to strangers just so they would survive, knowing that with almost absolute certainty, they would not be told where they were and that they might never see them again. His parents were the fourth members of his family to disappear from his life.

Years later, especially when his grandchildren reached the age of five, the age at which he said goodbye to his parents, Shaul would watch them and wonder what he'd felt at that moment, but he had no answer. His every traumatic memory had been buried, even though we know that five-year-old children can store experiences from that age in their subconscious memory.

Watching his grandchildren navigating the world at that age and so attached to their parents, he wondered how they would react if they were suddenly torn from their arms, told that they have to change their names, instructed to speak a different language, to forget their past, and were taken someplace unsympathetic and cold. As a young child, he may have explained to himself that he had to do as he was told because there were bad Germans outside, and that he simply had to obey her.

Two days later, Regina was taken into hiding. She didn't want to leave Perla, who was weak, but she insisted and repeated, "I don't know if I'll live, but you have to take care of Charlie."

She, too, didn't have time to say goodbye to her father, who was at the sweatshop, although for the rest of her life, the worst memory of that day remained of her mother, whom she left on her own in their apartment without a single child by her side, and whenever she talked about it, she would cry. She would also think about her father, who came home in the evening after a grueling day at work and found himself without his young children to light up his life—Regina, so lively and resourceful, and smiling, giggling Charlie. She hoped that he wasn't thinking already then that he would never see them again and that his end was approaching.

Decades after they were separated, when Charlie was already a father and grandfather himself, he would understand how pure, sublime and powerful his mother's love was, giving him up in that way; how deeply she loved him at that moment, when she handed him over to a trustworthy stranger. And although she'd be sent to the gas chambers only weeks later, after that unbearably difficult separation from her beloved son, she must have wished to die right then and there.

Almost anyone can bring children into the world, but not every mother is willing to sacrifice her own happiness for her children, and to repress her desires, longing and every expression of her own inner self in order to give them a chance for the future.

And perhaps because of this, although at the time no one explained to him why he was fated to live without his mother at such a tender age, Charlie could feel Perla's deep love for him, and could hold it hidden and free forever in his heart.

Charlie Hilsberg was given a new name and a secret code. His new name was Charles van Bergen, and his code number was CDJ.0423.

He was taken directly to the family health center in Nil-Saint-Vincent on the outskirts of Brussels, where he stayed for a few weeks.

WINTER 1943—MADAME MARTINE

A tall soldier in long shiny boots and an SS uniform walked into Madame Martine's apartment on Boondael Road in the Ixelles neighborhood. It was precisely those shiny black boots that caught Charlie's attention, perhaps because every time he'd heard the familiar loud tapping of military boots on the street near their home, he would notice his mother and sister cringing in fear. But the soldier with the noisy heels, who was planning to gain favor with the mistress of the house mistakenly thought that Charlie—now Charles Van Bergen—was her son, so he didn't aim his weapon at him. Instead, he smiled broadly, threw him in the air and laughed.

Charlie wanted to tell his mother that there was no need to be afraid of the men with the boots, but his mother was far away, and he didn't know when he would see her again. She had disappeared so suddenly from his life. Andree had fetched him from the family health center, not his mother, and she had brought him to Madame Martine's cold and strange ground-floor apartment and left him there without explaining why. But maybe she did explain, he couldn't recall. He didn't understand why he had to change his name and why he was forbidden from speaking Yiddish. He learned a little French at the family health center, but he wasn't sure of it, so he usually chose to remain silent. The mistress of the house didn't treat him kindly and compassionately, and he didn't understand why most of the time she wouldn't let him go outside. He ate mostly potato peels (although we should note that food was in short supply all over Belgium). She shouted at him and gave him chores to do, mainly cleaning. As such, even the fleeting touch of the Nazi officer, even the laughter of that uniformed man, made little Charlie less despondent. Later, Charlie would try to recreate what he'd felt then, but everything would be hidden behind an opaque black screen.

Because what can a five-year-old boy understand and then remember from those scary, lonely and cold days...of the apartment he was sneaked into in order to save him from the predatory grip of soldiers like the one who played with him so affectionately? Did he understand already then that evil has two sides to it? That the Nazi officer, who may have shot an elderly Jewish woman only two hours before, simply because she moved along the line too slowly for him, would play so tenderly with his son when he got home and then listen to a Beethoven symphony, his eyes gleaming with emotion. Could he have understood the contradiction in Madame Martine's behavior, who on the one hand treated him so harshly and often let him go hungry, while on the other hand was brave and moral enough to hide him, a Jewish boy, in her home, which was infested with German officers, and by doing so, save his life?

A few words about Madame Martine. Charlie remembered her vaguely as a pretty woman—her eyes were blue, and her hair was light and wavy. Her husband was recruited by the Germans to work and she offered her hospitality to the German officers who made regular pilgrimages to her apartment. Charlie had a few flashbacks from that period, which he sometimes wondered how real they were. One involved a loud, drunken argument between two German officers, which remained engraved in his memory. Both men wanted to get into Madame Martine's bed. There is no doubt that Madame Martine's daring behavior with the German officers could have put Charlie's life and the lives of the two other Jewish children she was hiding in danger. Charlie had only vague memories of the other children, and he never managed to trace them.

At only five-and-a-half, he was already certain of one important thing: he had to be alert and on his guard at all times, because life itself was unpredictable and anything could change in a flash. He was not allowed to speak Yiddish—his mother tongue—and he had to remember to speak only French. He was not to make a sound when he cried, or to even shed a tear—it would attract attention. He was not allowed to play with children outside because it was dangerous. Most importantly, he was forbidden from making any noise.

Such a high level of awareness could have benefited him, if it had not penetrated his soft consciousness in the form of trauma, with its many repercussions. Being a sensitive and intelligent child, Charlie's great fortune was that he spent his first five years with his parents before being separated from them forever, and they were wonderful, formative and critical years. His parents enveloped him in so much warmth and love that he could stay warm from their light throughout the other, cold and harsh years that would come later. They formed a solid foundation for him that helped him withstand the mental and physical hardship that followed.

He had no toys, he couldn't run about on the street, and he did not receive any of the enrichment that young children ordinarily receive.

Charlie's missed kindergarten years turned into missed school years. Only sometimes, when he was allowed to, he would sit on the doorstep and silently look at the street and people passing by, waiting for only one thing: to see his sister.

Regina had been luckier and was placed with nice people, a police inspector by the name of van Volden, on a street near to his.

They introduced her to their visitors as their niece. Since she was brave and had an Aryan appearance, she would go out but wonder how life could continue as usual while she and her family were suffering so.

Every few days, Regina would arrange to meet Charlie at the intersection between their two streets. She would bring him a block of chocolate or candy or some other treat, which Madame Martine never gave him.

Once, Regina was very daring and took Charlie to the cinema. They could have been caught, of course, but Regina took his hand and walked nonchalantly to the ticket booth, and from there into the dark cinema. She wanted her little brother to feel like any other normal child in the world, at least for a few hours.

When the film ended, she hugged him and said, "We need to go home now."

"*Vi iz heim*?" Charlie asked in Yiddish. "Where is home?"

He wasn't sure if she meant the home he'd grown up in with his parents, or the apartment he was living in now. Regina's heart went out to him. "To Madame Martine," she said sadly, stroking his hair.

A year later, Regina's relationship with van Volden's wife deteriorated when she wanted her to convert to Christianity, and she asked the Jewish underground member to transfer her to another family, the Rousseau family. The man was a cartographer, and she would help him. She was introduced to strangers as a Christian orphan. During her time with them, she lost contact with Charlie, until the end of 1944, when Belgium was liberated.

It was the fifth time that someone had disappeared from his life.

TRANSPORT NO. 20

On April 18, 1943, while their five-and-a-half-year-old son was learning how to live without basic human needs that every child has for food, warmth, and parental love, two Nazi officers burst into the home of Moshe and Perla Hilsberg, after they were informed on.

They had managed to hide in their apartment for just a few weeks. Perla was now weaker and even more ill. She'd heard nothing from Israel since he'd left, and after Marcel and Tola were taken to the camps, her heart couldn't bear that last separation from Charlie, her pride and joy, or from Regina, who was such a devoted and kind daughter. They lived in constant fear in their apartment, they were running out of food and it was dangerous to go out.

They were at least together at home, supporting and comforting each other, but even those moments of grace ended that miserable morning in April.

Perla was lying in bed when they heard someone banging on their door, a sound they had heard before, when their neighbors were raided.

"Faster, I don't have time for you," the SS soldier shouted at Perla, who was shaking and could barely get up. Moshe supported her.

The concierge looked at them, her face terrified and full of sorrow. Moshe nodded to her almost imperceptibly, and she blinked quickly, perhaps because of the tension, or maybe because of the tears threatening to well up in her eyes.

Before they boarded a truck to take them to the Dossin camp in the city of Mechelen, Moshe looked up at the free sky for last time and tried to breathe in what he saw and felt. He thought about the fact that the Nazis were waging two different wars: one visible, with aerial bombardments, battles, bleeding wounds, invasions and losses; and another, hidden, degrading war of mass murder against people without the means to defend themselves. And how ironic, he thought, that those red night skies of aerial bombardments also covered the camp they were now being taken to with their gray clouds. He wondered if he would get to see Marcel, not knowing that Marcel had been brutally killed by lethal injection after almost starving to death, and that a similar death was awaiting him, too.

The next day was April 19, the day that the Warsaw ghetto uprising began. It was also the day that the Germans transported them in long railway cars to their final destination, Auschwitz. Moshe and Perla, along with another 1,631 Jewish men, women and children were put on Transport No.20. It was the first train that used freight cars and it had barbed wire on the windows to make it hard for the prisoners to escape during the trip.

They were crammed in like animals and there was hardly any air. Their car was quiet. No one cried or shouted, although they guessed where they were going.

One of the cars contained 19 prisoners from a special list, and they were to be executed immediately upon arrival at the camp. Why? Because they belonged to the underground or had previously tried to escape from another train taking them to the camps. Their car was one before the last, which was for the guards. Perla and Moshe were in the front car. Perla was burning up with fever and Moshe stood up, arranged his small spot for her to lie down, and went to stand in another corner of the car.

It was ten o'clock in the evening when three young men on bicycles—Youra Livchitz, Robert Maistriau and Jean Franklemon from the Belgian resistance movement—rode toward the outskirts of Brussels. They carried a pistol, a lantern, red paper, and 50-Franc notes. They pedaled vigorously along the tracks in a secluded, rural area between Mechelen and Leuven.

The area was ideal for their mission, far from any city center and on a bend surrounded by thick vegetation.

Then, when the train switched to the track to Leuven, between the towns of Boortmeerbeek and Haacht, it suddenly stopped.

The reason for the unexpected stop: the three brave young men had covered the lantern with red paper to make it look like a danger signal, which made the driver think that there was a hazard on the track.

It was a rare and courageous operation that had never been used against the Germans before. Using the flashlight and a knife, they tried to cut the barbed wire used to close the cars. They could hear loud thumping, shouting, gunshots all around them, and then the cry, "Quick! Jump now!"

When the train stopped, Robert Maistriau, who was carrying their only gun, broke into Moshe and Perla's car and told everyone to jump out and save themselves. The gun contained only six bullets.

There was great commotion all around. Seventeen prisoners jumped out of their car, as many others were doing from the other cars, despite the barbed wire. The Nazis, who at first were confused and had no idea what was happening, finally understood to their great astonishment that it was a rescue operation and they started shooting at the fugitives.

Moshe's friend, a friend of the family, prepared to jump and called him to jump out with him. Perla also kept saying, "Moshe, jump, jump!" He took a long look at his beloved wife and saw that she couldn't possibly jump out, even with his help. She was simply too weak and ill.

He grabbed his friend's shoulder and said, "You jump, I can't leave Perla on her own here. I'm not leaving her, do you understand?"

His friend looked at him in surprise, gave him a quick hug and jumped off the train. After the war, he met Regina, told her his story, his voice wavering as he described that chilling moment of love and devotion.

The three young fighters quickly handed the cash out to the prisoners who had made it off the train and instructed them to disappear quickly. They themselves got back on their bikes and sped away under the cover of darkness. These men had helped 231 people to escape. Of these, 90 were captured and loaded onto another transport, 26 people were killed, and 115 managed to escape, two of them from the car marked for immediate death.

After the commotion subsided, the train continued its journey.

On April 22, Transport No. 20 arrived at the Auschwitz-Birkenau camp.

2003– THE TRUTH IS REVEALED IN AUSCHWITZ

Shaul Harel would find out what happened to his brother and father only sixty years later, when he visited the Auschwitz extermination camp and learned how they had died.

It was May 2003, and Shaul, now the President of the International Child Neurology Association, had been invited by the Polish Child Neurology Association to address an international conference being held in Warsaw. Until then, he'd avoided facing his past. All he knew was that his parents, brother Marcel and sister Tola had perished in Auschwitz, and he also had records of the transport and car they were in (the Germans being a very orderly people). He had mixed feelings about visiting Poland. Although his family was of Polish origin, it was also where his parents, brother and sister had been murdered. He was going to refuse the invitation but changed his mind and agreed to give a talk but asked them to arrange a tour of Auschwitz for him and other visitors.

The day that he and Dalia went to Auschwitz with the group was gray and gloomy, as if preparing them for what they were in for. Each buried in their own thoughts and emotions, no one uttered a word throughout the difficult and emotionally charged tour around the barracks. At the beginning of the tour, Shaul gave his family's details to one of the guides and asked her to find out what had happened to them. About an hour later, she appeared holding two documents, both death certificates. Shaul looked at them and his face turned as white as a sheet.

The first death certificate stated:

Name of the Deceased—Mordcha (Marcel) Hilsberg.

Age—18

Date of death—7 October 1942 (i.e., a few months after Marcel arrived in Auschwitz.)

Cause of Death—extreme exhaustion.

It was signed by Prof. Johann Paul Kremer.

Nr. 33963/1942   (935)   C¹

Auschwitz, den 7. Oktober _____ 19 4

D er Arbeiter Mordcha Hilsberg _____

_____ mosaisch _____

wohnhaft Brüssel, rue Montenegro 37 A _____

ist am 1. Oktober 1942 _____ um —13— Uhr — 00 — Minuten

in Auschwitz, Kasernenstrasse _____ verstorben.

D er Verstorbene war geboren am 15. Juli 1924 _____

in Warschau _____

(Standesamt _____ Nr. _____)

Vater: Mosek Hilsberg, wohnhaft in Brüssel _____

Mutter: Perla Hilsberg geborene Rotblatt, wohnhaft in _____

Brüssel _____

D Verstorbene war nicht verheiratet _____

Eingetragen auf mündliche — schriftliche Anzeige des Arztes Doktor der

Medizin Kremer in Auschwitz vom 1. Oktober 1942 _____

D Anzeigende _____

Vorgelesen, genehmigt und unterschrieben.

Die Übereinstimmung mit dem
Erstbuch wird beglaubigt.

Auschwitz, den 7. 10. 1942

Der Standesbeamte
In Vertretung

Der Standesbeamte
In Vertretung
Quakernack

Todesursache: Darmkatarrh bei Körperschwäche

Marcel's (Mordcha's) death certificate

His father Moshe's death certificate was also issued by the clinic, and the cause of death was the same: extreme exhaustion. It was dated August 1943, about three months after they arrived in Auschwitz.

Shaul and Dalia were horrified and stunned. Since when did the Germans bother to issue death certificates for the people they killed, and how could Moshe and Marcel have died in the same way? After all, they murdered millions in Auschwitz-Birkenau without anyone bothering to report them. Indeed, the guide who gave them the information apologized for not having any information regarding Shaul's mother, Perla, or his sister, Tola, as they were probably taken immediately to the gas chambers.

That night, when Shaul again saw the mysterious shadows that sometimes haunted him in his dreams, he realized that he was envisioning his father wrapping him under his prayer shawl in the synagogue, and his handsome brother galloping around the house with him on his sturdy shoulders when he was still a happy two-year-old toddler.

The flickering image of his brother carrying him on his shoulders had remained in Shaul's mind over the years, and for many years he deceived himself that perhaps Marcel, who was young and strong, had managed to survive; that perhaps he fled to Russia and couldn't contact the family; or, thinking that his entire family had perished, he had moved to another country without trying to contact his relatives. He was so self-delusional that in the mid-1990s, he found himself dining at the Four Seasons restaurant in New York with a man named Marshall Hilsberg, who at the time was the president of the well-known department store chain Lord & Taylor. Shaul contacted him because he thought that his name might once have been Marcel Hilsberg and that he changed his name to Marshall Hilsberg. It turned out that Marshall Hilsberg was a distant relative of Shaul's, and that they were linked through the renowned American musician Alexander Hilsberg, but no more than that.

And now here, in Auschwitz, in the most random of ways, the truth hit him in the face: his strong brother had died in Auschwitz from extreme exhaustion, and some doctor had even bothered to report his death.

Only when Dalia and Shaul returned to Israel, searched the Internet and went through the book *Anatomy of the Auschwitz Death Camp*[1] with a fine-tooth comb, they learned about Johann Paul Kremer—a physician who served as Mengele's deputy and who used Auschwitz as a research site for cruel experiments.

Johann Paul Kremer was born in 1883 in the city of Stelberg. In the early 1930s, he was a professor of anatomy at Münster University. In 1932, he joined the Nazi party and in 1934, he joined the SS. He was the only professor to serve as a doctor for the SS. He performed experiments in starvation and extreme exhaustion, and when his victims were actively dying, he would put them on his operating table, check their weight and order the SS medic to inject phenol into their hearts (death by phenol injection was the most common form of medical murder in Auschwitz). Then the professor would take biopsies of the victim's various organs and send them to Berlin to test the effect of hunger on the human body. Kremer was in Auschwitz from August 30, 1942 until November 18, 1942 and he took part in the selections. He was also present at the executions. He kept a diary of his experiences in Auschwitz, in which he described shocking scenes and stated that "Dante's Inferno seems to me almost a comedy compared to this." He also agreed with one of the military surgeon's description that they were located in the "anus mundi" (the anus of the world). At the same time, he didn't forget to mention his great pleasure from the various dishes of the hearty meals he was served. This is one of the most shocking (and rare) testimonies given from the point of view of the victimizer, and it has been quoted in books about the Holocaust, such as *Nazi Germany And the Jews: The Years of Extermination: 1939-1945* by Prof. Saul Friedlander.

---

1   Published by the United States Holocaust Memorial Museum, edited by Israel Guttman and Michael Berenbaum

And what happened to Johann Paul Kremer, who was personally responsible for murdering dozens of people? He was arrested in August 1945 and was sentenced to death in December 1947. He was meant to be executed in 1948, but his sentence was later commuted to life imprisonment, and ten years later, he was released due to his "extreme old age of 65," after which he lived peacefully in the Federal Republic of Germany. He was put on trial again for participating in two murders, but the German court ruled that the time he had already served in the Polish prison had "atoned him" for his actions. He was even a witness at the famous Frankfurt Auschwitz trials in 1964 and died in his sleep in 1965 at almost 82 years old.

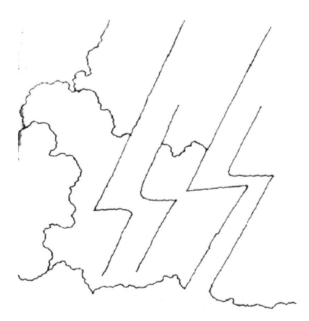

JOURNAL
de Johann Paul Kremer

1944—THE RULLAERT FAMILY

On one of the inspection rounds made by a member of the Belgian underground, she came to see how Charlie was doing with Madame Martine and reached the conclusion that his life was in danger.

The fact that there were always German soldiers hanging was of great concern to the heads of the CDJ and they decided that he had to be moved to another home. One day, when Charlie was already six-and-a-half years old, they came to take him to another Belgian family—the Rullaert family, who lived at 7 Rue de la Gouttiere.

For the second time in his short life, Charlie was uprooted and taken from the people taking care of him, even if this time it was from a bitter and loveless woman. Again, he had to adjust to a new environment and to strangers.

The Rullaert family lived too far from the home where his sister Regina was hidden. Not only that, but Regina had also been moved and they could no longer see each other. Thus, Charlie was left on his own for a long time.

The Rullaerts had no children. The woman, whose name was Lucy, was a large woman who behaved as aggressively as a man and had a stall where she sold French fries in a place called Coal Square. Her husband, a tram driver, was a thin, tall and quiet man. Despite their incessant quarrels, they treated Charlie better than Madame Martine had. They didn't make him work or let him go hungry. But here, too, he couldn't go outside to play because of the danger of informants, and here, too, he didn't receive the true love that all children need to develop.

In his autobiographical book, the psychiatrist Boris Sirolnik, who was also hidden as a child during World War II, explained that the memories of young children who experienced such trauma return later like shards that form a sequence, which their adult mind organizes. Thus, they can create coherence from that sequence...but not always. Sometimes, the memories remain as detached as shredded slivers of cloth that can't be reattached to form one complete dress.

Perhaps that is why, when many years later Shaul Harel struggled to recall the time he spent with the Rullaert family, he would mainly remember Mr. Rullaert sitting submissively in a tub full of water, naked as the day he was born while his oversized wife washed his hair, ordering him not to move. She would scrub his body so furiously that sometimes he would scream.

Madame Rullaert was not a bad woman, especially not to the child she'd taken into her care. Still, quite frequently, when she was annoyed and lost control of her emotions, she would pick a particularly loud argument with her husband, who would stand like a thin silhouette in the corner of the kitchen. To add icing on the cake, she would pick up a few plates and hurl them at his head. This memory was also firmly engraved in Charlie's mind.

The Rullaerts were religious, and he had to learn and memorize prayers and psalms. Every Sunday they would dress Charlie in his finer clothes, and he would attend the local church services with them. The images of singing in the church choir also remained engraved in his memory.

Although he had already passed the age of six, naturally he didn't go to school and he forgot that he was Jewish.

2013—WHO DID THE RULLAERT FAMILY REALLY HIDE?

It was many years later, when he met Andree Geulen, that Shaul learned that he'd been hidden by the Rullaert family. Meanwhile, Andree had received the Righteous Among the Nations award for her blessed work for the children of Belgium during the war.

His winding path had been recorded in the meticulous notes that she still had in her possession: the names of the families and places where he'd been hidden during the war. From these notes, Shaul learned that as of February 1943, he was hidden by Madame Martine, and about a year later, he was moved to the Rullaert family.

It was 68 years later, in March 2012, that he discovered a different truth.

In October 2009, Shaul and his wife Dalia's film, *Les Enfants Sans Ombre* (*Children Without a Shadow*) was screened for the first time at Yad Vashem, the World Holocaust Remembrance Center, and at the Museum of the Jewish People at Beit Hatfutsot. The film was produced by the Darden brothers and Belgian television, and was directed by Bernard Balteau, a Belgian journalist and director. The film tells Shaul's (Charlie's) story, as well as the story of the other rescued Jewish children of Belgium. The film has since been screened a number of times on Belgian television.

In March 2012, the film was screened at the Holocaust Museum in Paris. Robert Fuks, Shaul's close friend back since their time at Lasne and at Profondsart (institutions where he lived after the war), received an excited phone call from his wife in Brussels. She told him that her good friend's neighbor had seen the film on Belgian television and had very emotionally told her that Shaul couldn't have been hidden with the Rullaert family at 7 Gouttiere Street, because she herself had been hidden there. Her name was Rullaert, and she claimed that there were no other children with her!

This news greatly troubled Shaul, and he tried to get hold of the woman to talk to her, but his attempts to see her were met insistent refusal. The woman, who was a few years older than him, refused to talk to him, especially about the Holocaust period. She was a widow who had recently lost her only daughter to cancer and had been left alone to care for two relatively young granddaughters.

In the end, he managed to persuade her to talk to him. The woman's story was fascinating and moving.

Dina was from a large family and she had many siblings. When she was 12 years old, the Germans raided their neighborhood and started loading the Jews onto trucks. She started walking to the truck with her mother, three brothers and a sister. Her mother walked ahead with the three boys, while she walked behind, holding her little five-year-old sister's hand. Incredibly, a German soldier saw them, and his heart went out to them. He pushed them aside towards a Belgian woman and shouted at her, "Why are you not looking after your children?"

She was stunned into silence, but her little sister didn't want to go. She tore her hand away from Dina and ran after her mother and brothers, shouting "Mami, Mami!" The Germans, of course, hurried to take her, and only she stood silent and stunned by the Belgian woman's side as she watched her family getting onto the truck. It was the last time she saw them. The Belgian woman hid her for two days at home, but she was afraid of the risk. Her neighbor from 7 Gouttiere Street was known to belong to the underground and to forge documents, and so she asked him to take her. He agreed to take Dina in, she was given his surname and renamed Therese Rullaert. Charlie was, in fact, supposed to be taken in by them after he was taken from Madame Martine's care. Since they were already hiding the girl, he asked his downstairs neighbors—the tram driver and his wife—to look after him. They agreed on condition that Charlie's formal residence would be with the Rullaert family and that they would be the underground's contact person. That way, they couldn't be held accountable for hiding a Jewish child. According to Dina, the couple's names were Julian and Lucy Mary de Neef. And that's how it turned out that the two hidden children had the same fictitious surname without ever meeting each other, because they spent all their time in hiding and couldn't go out to play.

Dina was so grateful to the Rullaerts for hiding her, that after the war and until she got married, she kept their name.

Over the years, it had often seemed to him that the shards of memory hidden in his mind (in the form of flashbacks) were just figments of his imagination, but Dina confirmed that a somewhat strange couple had lived on the ground floor—a skinny tram driver and his fleshy wife. Her nickname was Fat Lucy and she used to sell pommes frites in Coal Square near Gouttiere Street. And yes, Lucy's hollering at her husband carried could be heard down the street. As it turned out, his memories were not wild imaginings that had invaded his mind.

THE END OF THE WAR BRINGS ISRAEL BACK

Neither the Catholic Church nor the Protestant Church took a public stand against the decrees and the deportation of the Jews, but they were active on all levels in helping the Jews, and their contribution to the rescue mission was enormous. Also, they usually didn't encourage any pressure on the children to convert while in hiding.

Towards the end of the war, Charlie was moved to a convent near the city of Leuven.

"I remember myself wearing a long white shirt and singing in church with other children in the choir," he told Yad Vashem in an interview.

How many identities could one child have before he even reached bar mitzvah age? How would the different identities affect his soul? The fact is, the hardships that Charlie went through were unable to weaken his spirit, perhaps because of the genes he inherited from his parents and grandparents, the love he was showered with as a child, or the role model he met at the orphanage he was sent to after the war—an extraordinary, warm counselor who took wonderful care of him and of the other boys.

Before that, however, he received a shocking surprise. His brother Israel, who had left home and enlisted in the French army when Shaul was two years old, had gone to war, been taken captive and then escaped and returned to fight. He heard that Shaul and Regina were the only members of the family to survive, and he first tracked Regina down. Israel wanted to know exactly what had happened to his family since that morning in 1939 when he left them and enlisted with burning faith in the French army. He wanted to hear all about the five years they had not seen each other; five long years in which he thought about his parents and siblings and prayed that they'd survive. Regina told him all about what he'd missed, and all about little Charlie.

"Your big brother is here to visit you," eight-year-old Charlie would be told when the war was over. He was weak and ill with a serious skin infection from the lice and fleas that he'd been infested with in one of his hiding places.

"What brother?" Charlie was surprised. "I don't have a brother. I only have one sister, Regina."

When Israel (Salek), a skinny but strong soldier in a British paratrooper's uniform adorned with medals came up to him in his bed, stepping lightly and smiling from under his light mustache, something melted in Charlie's heart and the memories slowly floated back.

But what is memory if not a deception? When asked to recall that reunion years later, the two brothers would remember it differently.

"I met you at a convent, and you were in terrible condition," Israel would tell Shaul. "And I immediately made sure you were taken to the hospital."

"That's not true," Shaul challenged Israel's recollection. "I remember that I was lying in the hospital and one of the nurses came up to me and told me that my big brother was there to see me. At the time, I still had no memory of you at all."

One thing they did agree on was that neither of them mentioned their parents. Israel knew what had happened to them, to their sister Tola and their brother Marcel. But Charlie didn't ask, and Israel had no intention of upsetting him. The future was still unclear, and they each quietly picked up the pieces and tried to move on.

Only when he grew up would Israel tell his brother about the upheavals he went through during the war, about the wounded people he saw, the shameful defeat of the French on the Maginot Line. He told him about when he was captured by the Germans and how he managed to escape only on his third attempt. He talked about the walking, hungry yet determined and confident that someone from the French underground would help him reach a safe destination. He would also tell him about how heroic the British were and how he admired for their determination. He was in their debt, and he joined them after escaping from German captivity, took part in the Battle of Normandy after parachuting across enemy lines and entering Brussels with them in October 1944.

It turned out that there were only a few survivors from the two large and extensive families, the Hilsberg and Rotblat families. Of Moshe's siblings, only his brother Mordechai, a renowned Yiddish actor, was left. Mordechai arrived in Palestine in the 1940s with what remained of the Polish army. Two of Moshe's cousins also made it through the war, one of whom survived because he converted to Christianity in his youth. Two of Moshe's nephews, Shmuel and Israel, survived by escaping through Siberia to Uzbekistan, where their parents, two sisters and a brother had starved to death. Shmuel and Israel immigrated to Israel after the war and settled on Kibbutz Gan Shmuel. Another of Moshe's relatives, his first cousin Motele Hilsberg, moved to Palestine in the early 1930s. He started a family and provided a warm shelter for the other remaining relatives when they first arrived in Palestine around and after the War of Independence, including Israel, Regina, and Charlie-Shaul.

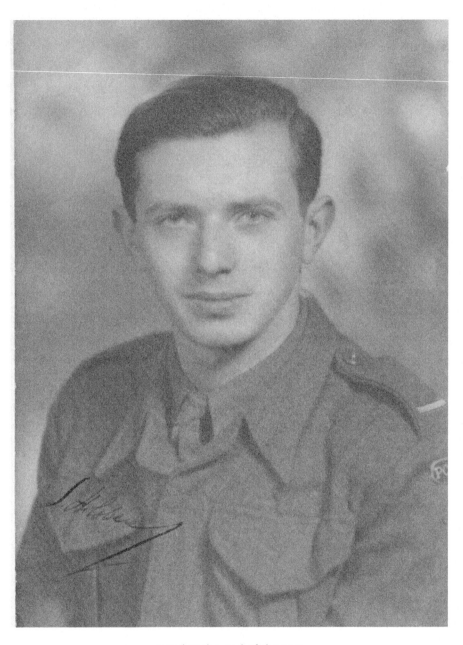

Israel at the end of the war

RECOVERY AND INTEGRATION IN ISRAEL

1945-1946—SIEGI, THE COUNSELOR WHO PUT A SMILE BACK ON CHARLIE'S FACE

The war was over.

The Germans had been defeated and the concentration and extermination camps liberated. The war was indeed over, but there was no cry of victory in the heart of the boy who would never again see his parents, Perla and Moshe Hilsberg, his beloved brother Marcel or his older sister, the beautiful Tola. Charlie believed himself to be all alone in the world and couldn't even remember his two surviving siblings.

He was transferred to an orphanage in Lasne, a pastoral town near Brussels, where other children like him, who'd been hidden during the war, were taken.

He has already learned that fate could be unkind, but now he would learn that sometimes magic happens, too. In his case, that magic went by the name of Siegi Hirsch. He was an Auschwitz survivor, tall and well-built, and had a thick black beard and a smile that stretched from ear to ear. Siegi defined himself as "a 20-year-old Tarzan."

As a child who had been moved from one loveless home to another, Charlie could have developed a natural and deep suspicion of new people that could have hung over him for the rest of his life. He could have lost the ability to form deep, intimate and significant relationships. But here, into the dark gaping abyss of his soul, entered Siegi carrying a powerful and healing light. He came and reminded the serious boy, who was already eight years old, how to laugh again.

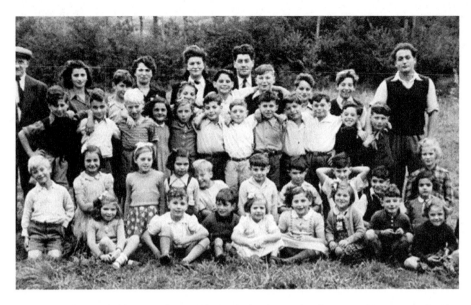

Siegi with the children: Robert Fuks and Charlie in the first standing row—third and fourth from the right

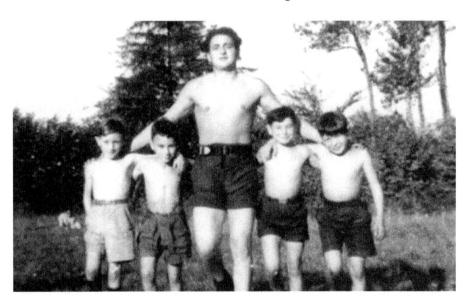

Siegi with children from Lasne. Charlie is on the far right, next to Robert Fuks

This was no trivial matter. Not only did his tears dry up during the war, but so did his laughter, which basically came from the same place—his sealed heart, which had helped him to survive. Releasing emotions had become extremely frightening.

Siegi, however, had secret weapons. He had love, and he had patience.

He kept a close eye on Charlie and the others at the peaceful orphanage. He could see their wounds, their vulnerability, the walls that they had built around their hearts, the restraint that was too mature for their age, their loneliness and pain, and the faith they had lost. And he knew what to do: find a remaining shred of hope in their little hearts, an intense desire to live, to simply live, in the most basic regular way... to exist. He knew that he had to take careful hold of that shred, hold it gently, and fish it out of the darkness; to feed them the bait of love and laughter, until they could hold their heads above water. Then, just like a tender mother, to hug them, love them, simply, unconditionally, fiercely and constantly.

He was a true and rare educator, with no theories or diplomas. He just knew that before he could teach the crushed, silent children, he had to first bring back a spark of passion and curiosity in their dead eyes. He used all of his artistic skills, put on theater performances with them so that they could express their deepest desires and emotions, which they'd had to suppress for so long. He exercised with them to strengthen their bodies, and as such, their minds, too. He played music for them and made them dance. Above all, he made them laugh. Who would have believed that those children, who throughout the war had learned to lay low, to be invisible, not to annoy anyone, not to demand anything, not to be loved, to cry without tears and to express almost no emotion—those children who were called *children of silence*, would suddenly start singing and dancing and go back to being children again, the way children should be?

He would go to the movies, usually to a double feature because that way, he could pay half the price, and come back to tell them the story. He had an excellent memory and a wonderful talent for drama, a wild imagination and a fine sense of humor, which made those nights wonderfully unforgettable for Charlie and his friends. He took them traveling around the world in their imaginations, had hair-raising adventures, identified with moving love stories and laughed at his ridiculous body language and the faces he made for them.

Siegi's magical stories replaced their nightmares.

Charlie, who later became Shaul, doesn't remember doing any schoolwork that year. He later learned that because there was no room for them at the local school in Lasne, the younger children stayed at the orphanage. Since he was eight years old, Charlie was one of the youngest, he, too, didn't attend regular school, which was freezing cold and sometimes boring. Instead, he was taught by Siegi, who even before he received an academic education realized that children could be taught more effectively through play.

No wonder then that he landed up becoming a well-known child and family therapist, a leading expert and guru of sorts in Europe. Thousands of therapists have made a pilgrimage to hear him talk about the theories and practices he developed.

It was at this institution that Charlie discovered the gift of friendship. His best friend at Lasne was Robert Fuks, and they remained close for years. They became even closer when Charlie revisited his past in the early 2000s. At Lasne, they were a gang of four smiley kids whose happiness is plain to see in the photos from that time. Siegi would eventually start calling them "My gang."

In the film about Shaul (Charlie) Harel, *Children without a Shadow*, Siegi said, "They were all obedient because they became very disciplined when they were in hiding. It wasn't a problem to organize them and give them structure, and there was no need for complex psychological theories."

They were children without a shadow, without a past, because being so young, their memories of home had been erased, and they also had to forget, because their identities had been changed. Many of them, like Charlie, even managed to erase their traumatic memories of the Holocaust, by embracing the rule: "We must forget that we have forgotten," or as Siegi said, "*La loi de l'oubli sur l'oubli.*"

In that post-war orphanage, they could begin to form a new shadow for themselves, with memories of sports, art, laughter, noise, commotion, life, a normal childhood and friendships. And memories of an extraordinary counselor, too, of course.

It's possible that these important moments in the life of young Charlie were an inspiration to Shaul, who would become a professor of pediatric neurology in great demand, well-known for the impressive way in which he examined the children that he diagnosed. His rooms would not be filled with the sounds of crying but with smiles and rolling laughter. Shaul always examined children while they're playing, including them so that they didn't feel that they were being examined or threatened in any way, or experiencing pain. Shaul would develop playful examination skills that were inspired by Siegi's example, and later by his teacher and master Prof. Nachum Boger, but that's another story. Shaul would travel around the world with two funny, floppy ragdolls and countless surprising and challenging little toys in his bag, which he would pick up on his travels around the world. He used these to examine the children's neurological responses and form clear and surprising diagnoses. He would know that his job was done when after being examined, the child would say to his or her parents, "You told me that we were going to the doctor, but all he did was play with me. That's no big deal!"

SIEGI—A TWIST IN THE PLOT

As a child, Shaul had revered Siegi, but he hadn't seen him since. In March of 2006, about 60 years after parting ways, the two of them met up, only to discover the chilling coincidence of fate.

After visiting Auschwitz, Shaul would occasionally travel to Belgium as part of his work with the International Child Neurology Association. He'd kept keen track of Siegi's career, but for some reason had never felt an urge to see him. Only when he started going back in time and remembering his past, only after meeting Andree Geulen and finding out what had happened to him during the war, did he feel that it was time to see Siegi as well.

They arranged to meet at the Crowne Plaza Hotel in Brussels at 7:30 in the evening. Siegi arrived at the hotel and asked at the reception for Charlie Hilsberg. Naturally, since Charlie had changed his name to Shaul Harel, there was no record of him on the hotel register. Shaul had forgotten to tell Siegi that he'd changed his name, and he was running a little late. Siegi was about to give up and leave when he arrived. They passed each other at the entrance and almost missed each other, but Shaul suddenly noticed his sturdy silhouette, which hadn't changed at all, even at the age of 82, and he shouted out, "Siegi! Siegi!"

They embraced, and since they both love to eat, went off to a well-known local restaurant, where they sat for an entire evening. They each talked about their past and told each other about their families and lives.

As a boy, Charlie never knew what had happened to Siegi before they met.

All he knew was that Siegi, just 19 years old, had survived the horrors of the Auschwitz extermination camp, but he was unaware of how much he had suffered during the war.

Siegi moved to Belgium from Berlin with his family in the late 1930s, perhaps because his family thought that Belgium would be friendlier to the Jews. Very quickly, however, just like Charlie's brother Marcel, he, too, was called up to enlist in the workcamps. He was transferred to Auschwitz on the first transport, along with thousands of other Jewish youths. He was immediately recruited to work in the log commando, felling trees and hauling them away. Since he was tall and strong, he managed to survive for quite some time, unlike many of the others subjected to starvation and hard physical labor.

It was not only his physical strength that sustained him during that horrifying period, but also his mental resilience and optimistic nature. His theatrical skills, along with his generosity and desire to cheer up people who were suffering, led him to set up a cabaret group in the camp. He himself was gifted with a strong and beautiful voice, and together with his friends, he would perform for the weak prisoners on a stage he built from wooden beams, as if it were in a famous theater. Every evening, he would end the show with a solo of the popular German song "Das Lied von der Krummen Lanke" in his perfect Berlin accent and mellifluous voice. This attracted the attention of the SS officers, including Prof. Kremer, the sadistic doctor who performed brutally cruel experiments on camp inmates. It was a very popular ballad in German cabarets and described a pair of lovers sitting on the bank of a river that meandered through the mountains.

Siegi, too, eventually became weak after contracting dysentery. Exhausted and pale, one day, when selecting the morning shift, the duty officer motioned to him to move over to the group destined for the crematoria. Siegi sipped his mug of thin, murky soup, his only food for the day, and naked as the day he was born, made his way to the truck, which was there to take that morning's selected group to their deaths.

Suddenly, the famous Prof. Kremer appeared, making them all tremor in fear, and began inspecting the people getting on the truck, like a zoologist examining the insects he'd just caught. Siegi was standing in the long line behind a Polish man who started begging for his life: "I'm a famous director, please don't send me there!" But his loud pleading was interrupted by a pistol shot. He fell to the ground in a pool of blood, which spread around his head. Prof. Kremer, who had just shot him in the head at zero range, glanced indifferently at the body laying at his feet.

Siegi held his breath and tried not to collapse. He was next in line, and Kremer's scrutinizing eyes flashed in recognition.

"Oh, you're that singer who sang the 'Das Lied von der Krummen Lanke'," he said. "My son also sings that song well," he added proudly. "No, you're not getting on this truck."

Dumbfounded and bewildered, Siegi was removed from the line and sent to work in the political prisoners' section, where the work was easier, and they received a little more food. And so Siegi survived until the end of the war.

The fact that he'd so miraculously survived drove him to give even more to others, and he decided to help the children who'd suffered during the war and been robbed of a normal childhood.

He decided to volunteer at the orphanage, where he gave Charlie and his friends inspiration and restored their faith in the goodness of life.

It was only that evening, 60 years later in the restaurant in Brussels, that they both learned the blood-curdling fact that Prof. Johann Paul Kremer, who'd caused the deaths of Shaul's brother and father, first by torture and eventually by phenol injection into their hearts, had also chosen to save Siegi in a momentary whim, and Siegi would later go on to save the soul of the boy Charlie Hilsberg.

1947-1949—PROFONDSART BOARDING SCHOOL

After a year in Lasne, Charlie was transferred to another home for Jewish children—a boarding school in Profondsart, which was sponsored by the Joint and where he would stay for the next two-and-a-half years. Was he resilient enough? Immune to being separated from his loved ones and to adapting to a new place where it was unclear how he would fit in? No one asked that question when Charlie was moved yet again to somewhere new.

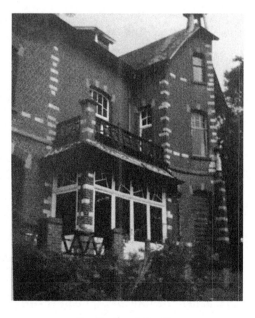

Profondsart Castle

It was a castle in the middle of the woods with a large terrace looking out. It had been converted into an orphanage by the Joint. Shaul remembers it as a pastoral place with a large courtyard covered with grass and nearby a swimming pool.

The yard was a hive of activity for the children, who were all Holocaust survivors like him. They climbed trees and swam in the pool. Charlie, who was an outstanding athlete, felt that he was growing stronger and beginning to take his place as a leader in the group. At the end of the yard, there was a warehouse where they could do handicrafts, and they devoted a great deal of time to this. The castle was located in a rural area on the outskirts Brussels. Every day, the Jewish children walked more than a mile to the mixed school in Limal, the nearest town, where Jews and Christians studied together. It wasn't the walk that the Jewish children found most difficult but the fact that even though the war was over, "normal" life had not yet erased the animosity planted in the hearts of some of the Christian boys in the area. Every morning, when they walked to school, a gang of bullies, peasants still full of hatred for the minority who had just been rescued from danger, would be waiting for them. They had a strong urge to beat up Charlie and his Jewish friends and would set up traps and ambushes for them. Once again, Charlie had to muster his fortitude in order to survive. The combination between his mental resilience and his physical strength had turned him into one of the leaders of the group. They did occasionally take beatings, but they fought back, and withstood the attacks with dignity.

After not having any real formal education, he began school at nine years old in Limal. Their teacher, Monsieur Froncee, was one of the people who shaped Charlie's future path, and he remains forever in his memory.

The class was rather strange: each line of desks constituted a separate class, and Monsieur Froncee taught them all. Although Charlie was supposed to be in fourth grade, he actually started from first grade, and finished a grade every two months, until he reached the fourth. In the next two years, he completed fifth and sixth grades.

Charlie was an outstanding student, and Monsieur Froncee liked and admired his new student. Despite the fact that he hadn't been to school before, his inherent curiosity had not been ruined by the years of isolation, and he diligently and joyfully swept through his studies. Most of all, Charlie remembered the thick tree that grew gloriously in the middle of the schoolyard, and the children climbing it during breaks, collecting acorns and throwing them at each other. When they had a penny in their pocket, they would go to the candy store across the road and buy themselves a treat. There is no doubt that the appreciation and warm feelings that Monsieur Froncee showed Charlie boosted his self-confidence.

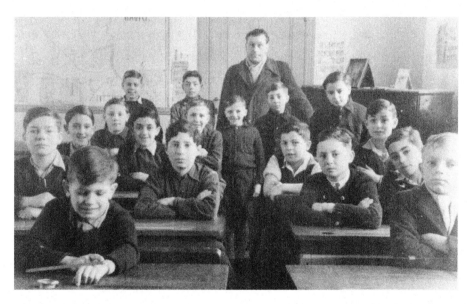

Shaul in Monsieur Froncee's class—second from the right in the third row

Close to 40 years later, in 1986, when Shaul was almost fifty, he took his family on a trip to Europe, including Belgium. He didn't take his children to visit his pre-war neighborhood in Brussels, but he really wanted to show them the school he attended. They were a big group: Shaul and Dalia, their three children, Tali, Ronit and Gil, who were in their teens, Dalia's mother Grandma

Yehudit, and Uncle Arie.

They arrived in Limal and find the school, which was still standing tall and unruined. The children were very excited to see the impressive building, which was still being used as a school, and the tree that their father told them was centuries old, with a pile of acorns on the ground under it. The candy store across the road was still there, and they were eager to buy candy in memory of those days. Suddenly, Dalia casually asked Shaul, "Do you think that Monsieur Froncee is still alive?"

Shaul doubted it. "It's been so many years," he said.

When they were ready to leave, Shaul saw an old man in the yard of a house by the school tending his potted plants. He got out of the car, went to talk to the man, and returned excited, saying, "That man told me that Monsieur Froncee is still alive, and he lives right at the end of the street!"

It was the middle of the day, not a good time to visit, but Shaul insisted. The whole big bunch of them went with him to the door and rang the doorbell. A young woman opened the door and Shaul asked, "Is Monsieur Froncee home? I was his student between 1947 and 1949."

The woman exclaimed excitedly, "Papa, Papa, come quickly, a former student has come to visit you."

Monsieur Froncee came to the door, and although Shaul's hair was now starting to go white, he immediately said, "You must be Charlie Hilsberg."

Monsieur Froncee was in his late 70s and was showing minor signs of Parkinson's disease, but he looked good, and his mind was sharp. The reunion was moving, and they reminisced. Monsieur Froncee's family had also been impacted by the war, and part of the family had perished in an Allied shelling, of all things. Monsieur Froncee's voice choked when he said that the height of his teaching career was the period in which he taught Holocaust orphans, who amazed him with how motivated they were.

Later, Froncee's daughter wrote the following to Shaul:

"Sometimes, a person regrets having only one child, and in his case, me, a daughter. But my father never felt that way because of the horrors of war. I'm sure that you remember him loving you more than a teacher loves his students. The most important thing for a 'father' is to be proud of his children and realize that neither time nor distance can damage their emotional bond. Thank you from the bottom of my heart for visiting him in the summer. He found meaning in life again after seeing you and your family."

BRUSSELS, 1949—DECIDING TO LEAVE BELGIUM

Perla and Moshe, Charlie's parents, had perished in the camps. But Perla's sister, her husband and their children had survived, thanks to their wealth and the button factory they owned. They apparently managed to bribe the right people and find a good, protected place to hide. In contrast, Charlie's family had only a slim chance of surviving, as they lacked financial means. Yes, even then money was an important factor in survival, although one certainly also had to be lucky. The sisters lost touch when the war broke out, and Perla didn't know where her sister and her sister's family were.

After the war, when Regina was 16, they took her in. Charlie, who was just seven years old when the war ended in Belgium, could have done with a warm and loving home, but for some reason, they didn't take him in, and he spent four years in orphanages. Regina didn't like living with her aunt and uncle. She didn't feel comfortable in their home. She spent most of her time doing housework and was not sent to school, even though she was a smart and intelligent girl. They never visited Charlie, perhaps because they were busy trying to make a living. Only every few months, he was sent to visit them in Brussels, and the highlight of his visits was the ice cream he ate at Bouquet Romain on Rue Neuve, a popular ice cream parlor in the 1940s.

One day, the beautiful Regina met a handsome brigade soldier by the name of Chaim Bernstein on the stairs of the Brussels stock exchange, and she decided to start a life with him, and after a while, to immigrate with him to Israel and start a family. They arrived in Israel at the end of the War of Independence and married soon after that. The ceremony was modest but warm, and they held it at Regina's relatives, Motele and Hindeleh Hilsberg. Motele (you may recall), was Moshe's cousin and was also in the tie manufacturing business. He and his wife Hindeleh immigrated to Israel as early as 1932 and had three children. They welcomed all the Hilsbergs with open arms, and to Charlie, they were his real uncle and aunt.

Charlie's older brother Israel moved to London after the war and studied at the School of Economics. As he'd been a soldier in the British Army, he received a scholarship, which was how he managed to fund his studies. Every so often, he would visit Regina and Charlie in Brussels. When the War of Independence broke out, he couldn't sit back without getting involved, so he enlisted in the Israeli Army. After all that he'd been through during World War II, which he came out of unscathed, he was severely wounded in the War of Independence, stayed in Israel and found work with the Belgian airline Sabena.

After Regina and Israel immigrated to Israel, each on their own, 12-year-old Charlie realized that he, too, belonged there. The Jewish organization that took care of orphans in Belgium, Aide aux Israelites Victims de la Guerre, or AIVG, also concluded that Charlie belonged in Israel with his siblings.

When Charlie's uncle heard that he was leaving, his feelings of guilt over allowing Charlie to be moved from orphanage to orphanage must have bothered him, because he called him over for a talk. "Why go to Israel, it's dangerous there? Stay here and I'll teach you the tricks of the button trade," he said. "Eventually, you'll become a work manager and make a good living for yourself." (He was about to hand the factory over to his son to run.)

And how surprised he was when Charlie politely shook his head and turned down his offer. For even before he knew what he would do when he grew up, it was clear to him that his ambitions didn't end with being an insignificant, even if it could make him wealthy, and that he was aiming for a more inspiring future. He may have missed a thriving career in buttons, but that's how Charlie was planning to end the 12-year chapter of his life in his country of birth, Belgium.

He had spent a little over five years with his warm family before the significant people in his life slowly began to abandon him: his older brother Israel, his middle brother Marcel, his sister Tola, and finally his parents and sister Regina. From then until the age of 12, he was moved to four hiding places and two orphanages. As an adult, he often asked himself if moving so often and having no close family for support had hurt him. Could he have possibly not been hurt by it, or did it make an emotional dent on him, which he would bear for the rest of his life? Would he become like everyone else?

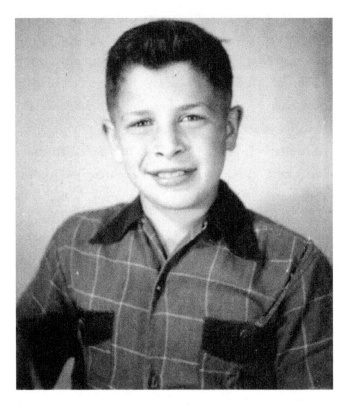

Shaul when he immigrated to Israel at the age of 12

LATE 1949–ANTWERP AND FROM THERE TO VILLA GABY IN MARSEILLE

The Youth Aliya movement had taken on the important job of rehabilitating young survivors by bringing them to Israel, sending them to kibbutzim or moshavim and integrating them in schools, which would help them to catch up with their studies.

Charlie was transferred to an orphanage in Antwerp where all the children immigrating to Israel on the same ship were staying

From the protective and warm walls of Profondsart, he moved to a more conservative orphanage for Jews that was cold and gloomy. It didn't have the green expanses of the previous home, only a paved courtyard without a single plant or even a swing or a slide to play on. They were dealt with rigidly and impersonally, and the head was alienated and distant. Luckily for Charlie, he was moved about two months later to a wonderful place that will always remain engraved in his memory—Villa Gaby in Marseille.

All the children from Youth Aliya were sent to Villa Gaby in Marseille for a few weeks, where they were given a short preparation before immigrating to Israel. In other words, they began to learn a little Hebrew, Israeli songs and dances and a little bit of Zionism. It was a happy time. In their free time, they would jump off the cliffs into the Mediterranean, and if they had a penny in their pocket, they would wander a while through the main streets of Marseille. Sometimes, they would go to the cinema and see a French action movie. Shaul remembers his craving for the juicy Marseille oranges, which he would make a hole in, pour sugar into and suck out their juice. To this day, he eats oranges in this wasteful way. They enjoyed their new freedom and the exciting status of being future immigrants to the Jewish state, a place where they believed they would never again fall into the hands of the murderers who took their parents and siblings and cousins from them. Everything was open and bright and full of hope for the new future.

NOVEMBER 1949—THE SHIP GALILA AND ARRIVING IN ISRAEL

Their new future was weeks away from where they were, and where they were right then was a rundown, very basic ship that was crowded to the point of suffocation. It was an old 1913 river ship that ZIM converted into a passenger ship to take immigrants to Israel, but it remained a river ship.

They crowded 200 children onto the rickety ship. The sanitary conditions were terrible, and naturally, there were no beds. The children had to sleep on the hard deck on makeshift blankets.

There was a terrible stench in the air, the food was awful and bland and Shaul and his friends, having nowhere to escape to, were miserable. As if that wasn't enough, the ship stopped on its way to Israel in the Port of Benghazi in Libya and picked up 250 families with children. The crowding was unbearable, and they suffered terribly. The days felt like weeks.

The deplorable conditions on the trip did have one special and unforgettable moment: it was seven in the morning, the sun was rising slowly in the sky when a wonderful and incredible sight appeared before the astonished eyes of the children and families who had dreamed of that moment. The shoreline of Haifa Bay slowly became visible and clear in a distance.

The blue waters of the Mediterranean kissed the brown land, leaving the passengers breathless. Their eyes twinkled with excitement as they looked in wonder at the Land of Israel, the Holy Land of the bible. They were no longer a minority in a foreign land, nor were they persecuted immigrants; they were proud citizens that were not ashamed or afraid to die just because they were Jewish. No wonder the Libyan immigrants were so emotionally moved that they knelt on the ground and kissed it, their eyes filled with tears. To this day, Shaul is moved whenever he flies home from abroad and sees Israel's coastline, which he always waits for with anticipation.

"I've come home," Charlie whispered to himself, wondering what his new life would be like.

NITZANIM

Funding for the campaign came from a generous donation from Romi Gold-muntz, a community leader and avid Zionist from Antwerp who made his fortune in the diamond business. He fled to London during the war, played a role in maintaining the Belgian government while in exile in England and helped to hide Jewish children.

He felt deeply for the children who found themselves orphans after the war, and he decided to donate money to the Youth Aliya organization.

Upon his arrival in Israel, Charlie's name was arbitrarily changed, as the authorities did that time, and Charlie David Hilsberg became Shaul Hilsberg.

Shaul and his friends, who like him were Belgian orphans and Holocaust survivors who had already been through too many upheavals in their short lives, arrived at the Sha'ar Ha'aliya Absorption Camp in Haifa, where they were sprayed with DDT, as was the norm in those days. Then they were scrubbed and thoroughly cleaned. It was here that he met up with Regina and her new husband Haim for the first time in Israel.

A few days later Shaul and his friends were accompanied to Nitzanim Youth Village by their school principal and a few of their counselors, who had come with them from Belgium. In 1949, the Jewish Agency's immigration depart-ment decided to establish a youth village where Kibbutz Nitzanim used to be, before it was conquered and destroyed by the Egyptians during the War of Independence. It was subsequently taken back by the Israelis. A team of educators was sent there, and the teachers and youths set themselves up in the old, damaged buildings from the Mandatory Palestine period. They ironically called the main building the Sheikh's House, the White House, or the Mansion. It was a two-story building with lots of rooms and balconies. The buildings had been destroyed during the War of Independence and the first new occupants of the Zionist Youth Village started to fix them up.

The original concept was wonderful: to take care of the youths and educate and prepare them for their new life in Israel. In practice, their reality was bleak. When Shaul and his friends arrived at Nitzanim, there were already two other groups of immigrants there: one from Morocco, and another from Turkey. The counselors couldn't control them and there was no fixed curriculum. Fights broke out between the various groups, none of the kids learned in an orderly fashion, and they did not yet speak Hebrew.

"Most of the time we ran around in the dunes," Shaul recalls. "There wasn't enough food, and we went to the wild orchards near the youth village to find edible fruit. We swam unattended in the sea and a few of the boys drowned. And the Sheikh's House, where we slept, didn't have an actual roof and the walls had been perforated by Egyptian bullets during the War of Independence."

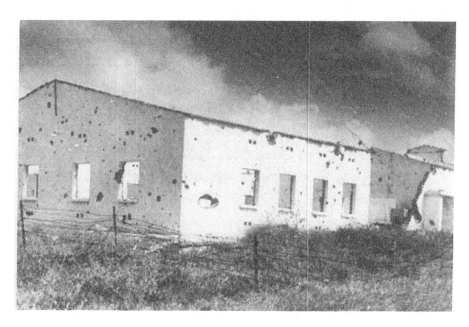

Nitzanim Ruins

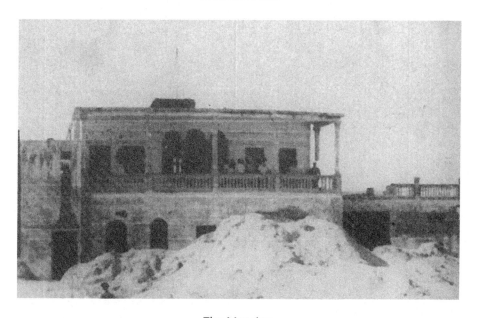

The Mansion

The building had not yet been properly renovated, and as it was early winter, the wind was cold and the rooms freezing. Shaul and his friends took no comfort in knowing that they could see the moon and stars in their new land. Despite their sense of freedom, they had nothing to do for hours, which only made the run-ins between the groups worse.

The only shimmer of light at the time was the Belgian group, which formed a close clique. This stopped them from feeling like strangers in their new country. They spoke to each other in French, their mother tongue, played a French card game called Belote, at which Shaul excelled. Basically, they did their best to survive the challenging year. Shaul continued to improve his leadership qualities and was one of the leaders of their clique.

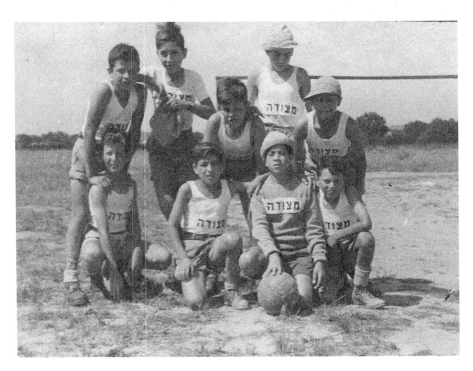

Shaul with a group of children at Nitzanim—Shaul is on the far left in the second row

Luckily for Shaul and his Belgian friends, after almost a year had passed, their Belgian patron, Romi Goldmuntz, decided to visit his proteges at Nitzanim. The youth village's management immediately went to work getting the place ready, they cleaned the Sheikh's House, and the children stood dressed in their smarter clothes holding flags. They waited for the distinguished guest to arrive, but for some reason, he decided not to visit that day, and instead arrived about a week later, when everything was normal again. When he arrived, he was astonished by the disorder and neglect and the children told him about the hunger, lack of schooling and the fights with the other groups.

He quickly called Moshe Kol, who was the head of Youth Aliya at the time and demanded in no uncertain terms to transfer the children immediately, without delay, to another youth village. Kol understood the way Goldmuntz felt and thought straight away of the Aloney Yitzchak Youth Village.

Shaul and many of his friends managed to survive the rather traumatic period at Nitzanim, but some of his other friends, who couldn't bear the situation, decided to leave the youth village and some even the country. No one looked for them. They slept on the streets and in deserted buildings. Some were arrested by the police and two eventually stowed away on a ship and made their way back to Belgium.

Only many years later did Shaul meet them, and to his surprise, one of them had become an anesthesiologist and dentist, and the other was a factory manager. They seemed to have come out of their past stronger.

ALONEY YITZCHAK

The children were sent by bus to Aloney Yitzchak, near the farming village of Givat Ada and Kibbutz Kfar Glikson, in a beautiful rural area near the hills of Samaria. They were taken to their rooms and everyone looked forward to meeting the well-mannered European group.

But after a year of being hooligans for all means and purposes, they were restless and went out at dawn to hunt, as they did at Nitzanim.

Aloney Yitzchak was run by a renowned educator with excellent pedagogical skills by the name of Yehiel Harif. He assembled all the students and told them that a group of very well-mannered and "refined" Belgian children had arrived, and they were to treat them accordingly. What he didn't know was that the "refined" Belgian children had caught all the fish in the ornamental pool by the dining room.

"When we talk about survival," Shaul explains, "not only DNA should be considered but also the severity and duration of any trauma, as well as the environment in which the child grows up afterward. The first five years are the most significant when it comes to a child's ability to survive in the years that follow (the ability to create trust, mental fortitude). Still, one must not forget that the environment in which the child lands up after the traumatic experience will in most cases predict the child's mental resilience, ability to succeed despite the traumas, and to catch up and bridge the gaps."

For example, it was very difficult for children of Holocaust survivors who could not function as parents because of the experiences they had during the war to recover later from past traumas. "Nitzanim," he adds, "was another blow to their ability to survive. I didn't even know how to read and write in Hebrew, and I was still speaking French with my friends when I was sent from there to Aloney Yitzchak. That move constituted a corrective and formative experience that made me, and my group feel that had an organizing hand to guide us, that there was someone to trust, and that we could finally become true Israelis."

There is no doubt that Aloney Yitzchak was a vastly different story from Nitzanim, and to this day it is known in Israel for its high level of education and the values it imparts to its students. It was spacious and beautiful. It was in a nature reserve with thousands of cyclamens that bloomed in the winter, and even then, the children were taught not to pick wildflowers. The spacious dining room stood at the top of the hill and Shaul nostalgically remembers that the food was incredibly delicious. It was a period of austerity, but the cooks used all their skills to serve the children delicious and nutritious food. The children's rooms were modest shacks, with four children per room, but the caregivers were motherly and warm, and in the evenings, they would sometimes come into the rooms to cover the children. There was a huge lawn by the dining hall where the groups of children would hang out together and play, by the ornamental fish pond that the Belgian children had raided on their first day.

By the time Shaul moved to Aloney Yitzchak in the late 1950s, he was already 13 years old. He hadn't had a bar mitzvah ceremony (and he hasn't had one to this day). He still didn't know Hebrew and he had a huge task ahead of him: to acquire a new language and catch up in his studies, as the only serious education that he'd received had been during his three years at Froncee in Belgium.

He was inspired to study by the mythological principal Yehiel Harif, who had taught at the Ben Shemen school. He had also taught Shimon Peres, who would later become the prime minister and then the president. He had no children of his own, and the children at the youth village served as a kind of substitute. He would often gather the kids in the evening and broaden their education beyond the curriculum, and the kids would lie on the rug in his house and listen eagerly to his lectures on history, the bible, Greek plays and more. Another of Aloney Yitzchak's founders and its first school principal, Gershon Bergson, worked alongside him. Gershon Bergson later moved up the ladder at the Ministry of Education where he reached a senior position.

That was how Shaul first learned proper Hebrew, and where he and his friends were exposed to all aspects of Israeli culture and life—the songs, the dances and the stories. They went on trips around the country. The youth village had a local newspaper and radio station, a folk dancing club and plenty of sports activities. Every Saturday afternoon, the children would tune into a program on the Kol Yisrael national radio station, which would play the songs that listeners requested.

The youth village felt like home and the youths were clearly willing to be absorbed quickly and to integrate. The days were divided in two: they studied half the day and worked at Aloney Yitzchak or on Kibbutz Kfar Glickson during the other half. The days were split according to the teachers' schedules. Shaul's favorite job was to lead the old, exhausted mule hitched to a rickety cart and collect bread from the bakery in Givat Ada. He would take the opportunity to nibble on some hot, fresh bread. His craving for bread was common knowledge.

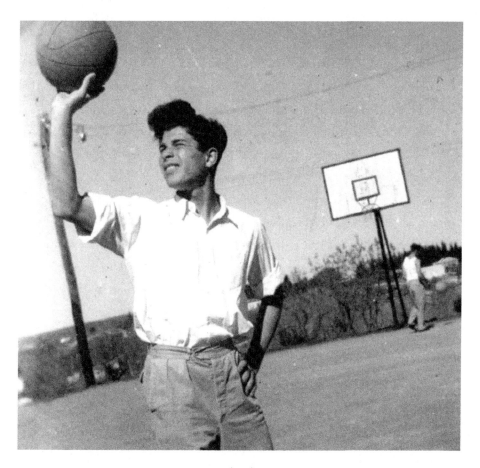

Shaul

All the kids played plenty of pranks, but the Belgians stood out in this area. There was a vegetable garden in the youth village, where one of the older instructors used to plant vegetables, including carrots. The carrots were juicy and tempting and the Belgian kids would find them, pull them out and eat them, leaving just the tops, which they would return to the vegetable beds. The instructor had no idea what to do and couldn't work out what mysterious disease was so cruelly attacking his carrots. He called in an expert agronomist, who examined the carrots and explained to him that no worm could eat the carrots so perfectly and leave just their tops intact, and that he should secretly watch his vegetable garden.

Those were happy times, times that gave them a boost in an educational atmosphere. Shaul began to grow attached to his new country and to feel that he belonged. He studied hard and the principal encouraged him.

The children were divided into groups, and Shaul belonged to the Shahar Group, in which he made friends, both younger and older. Some of the teens paired off, and yes, Shaul also met his first girlfriend, Shoshana.

Sometimes, during school vacations and on weekends, Shaul would occasionally visit Regina and Israel. Regina lived in Ra'anana and had two children, Pnina (Perla in Hebrew) and Moshe, who were named after their parents. Her apartment was rather cramped, and whenever Shaul came to visit, her husband Haim would have to sleep in the bathroom. Still, he was always received with open arms and a smile. In those days, strolling up and down Ahuza Street and buying light refreshments at the Tnuva restaurant. It was considered a night out on the town. They didn't have much money.

Israel, although already over 30, was still single and would occasionally invite Shaul to stay over at his basic apartment in Tel Aviv and take him to a movie. There was a 15-year age difference between them.

At the age of 32, Israel found the love of his life, Annie, a Holocaust survivor from Belgium, who, after a quick one-week courtship, agreed to share a life with him and immigrate to Israel. They started a family and had two children of their own, Moshe and Daphna. Shaul loved to visit his nieces and nephews and to take them for walks, hang out on the beach with them and carry them on his shoulders, and they enjoyed having a young and energetic uncle.

THE ARMY, AN INJURY
AND THE PURSUIT
OF MEDICAL STUDIES

A MATRICULATION CERTIFICATE AGAINST ALL ODDS

There is no doubt that Shaul's time at Aloney Yitzchak contributed greatly to his integration in Israel and boosted his self-confidence. He was lucky to spend five years at a school where all the children were Holocaust survivors, and most of them orphans. The homogeneity of the students, who the tough farmers of nearby Givat Ada called "the elite of the Holocaust," made it possible for them to forge their way without frustrating confrontations with born and bred Israelis, or sabras, as they were called. That was what usually happened on kibbutzim. Those confrontations, some survivors have claimed, sometimes reduced the refugee children's self-confidence and cut them down. Only when Shaul was drafted into the army would he have to deal with such issues, but in the meantime, he had already acquired all the self-confidence he needed.

As wonderful as it was, Aloney Yitzchak had one drawback: the school did not submit its students to take matriculation exams.

The path for Shaul's class was fixed and predetermined, and no one thought of questioning it. The kids were expected to finish school and enlist in the pioneering Nahal Brigade infantry, with a Zionist youth movement group, called a *garin*. The garin would do part of their army duty on a kibbutz, with the aim of becoming members.

Shaul had other plans. He felt that he wasn't suited to be a kibbutznik, and he wanted to be able to continue his studies at university.

It's no small matter for an 18-year-old orphaned immigrant whose first language wasn't Hebrew and who had experienced such difficulties as a child to go against the norm and decide to obtain his high school diploma. Where did this drive come from?

Shaul insisted.

Using his charisma and determination, he managed to convince four of his classmates, including Shaul Yatziv, Arie Shtro and Ephraim Berkowitz, who later continued with him to university, that they should do their matriculation exams, even if they had to postpone the army for a short while. This caused an uproar among their fellow students. All the other kids from their year were angry with them for not wanting to serve their country or to join a garin in the conventional way and work the land. Some of them treated them with contempt and called them "that bunch of professors."

Now the question remained as to who could approve such a thing, and what school they would attend.

Shaul decided to turn to Yehiel Harif.

Yehiel Harif was admired and looked up to not only by his students but also by people in key positions in education. Therefore, when Shaul asked for his help in postponing their induction by six months so that they could sit for external matriculation exams, he immediately agreed. He spoke to his personal friend, Moshe Kol, who was the former head of Youth Aliya and was now the chairman of the Progressive Party. Kol came to their rescue again and helped them to postpone their induction by a few months.

There were no suitable teachers at Aloney Yitzchak, and the boys also had to fund their extended stay there.

Harif solved the problem by making an agreement with them: they would work half of each day at the youth village, and he himself would teach them and prepare them for their matriculation exams in literature, history and bible. Talia, the wife of the head counselor, was American, so he put her in charge of their English lessons, and another friend of his from Aloney Yitzchak who knew math prepared them for their math exam. Naturally, their studies were not orderly, so they relied on the fact that Yehiel Harif was quite the polymath. They gathered every evening on the carpet in his humble house, and Shifra, Harif's wife, provided them with a constant supply of tea and biscuits. Harif would interpret the bible for them, analyze Greek tragedies, explain important historical events and more.

That was how the five friends prepared for their matriculation exams. Their grades weren't great to say the least, but they still received their high school diplomas.

HEY, YOU, YOU REFUGEE, YOU BAR OF SOAP!

With terribly flat feet and pain when walking, Shaul enlisted in the army. And since his class from Aloney Yitzchak had already enlisted in the Nahal garin six months earlier, he joined another. It was an elitist garin from Jerusalem of mostly Israeli-born soldiers. The army was supposed to mark the final chapter of his full integration into Israeli society, but these optimistic expectations were suddenly dashed when he met the Israeli group. Since all the kids at Aloney Yitzchak were Holocaust refugees, Shaul had never felt socially alienated from them, but in the army, he encountered the rough and somewhat arrogant sabras for the first time, who condescendingly scrutinized the new immigrants. They looked down on them for being too pale, speaking poor Hebrew and having parents who went like sheep to the slaughter. Now and then, he would even hear them call him "the refugee" or by the horrifying nickname "soap," which the Germans were rumored to make from their victims' body fat.

For a while, Shaul felt as helpless as he'd felt when in hiding, without his parents or siblings or a loving touch. He felt lonely because he was the only soldier in the garin who was a refugee. This time, it was not his Jewishness that worked against him, but his European origins.

It was a slap in the face, and it worried him: Would he ever belong? Would he always be different? Would he always have to try to catch up in order to be like everyone else?

"It seemed to me that I was already considered Israeli in every possible way," he recalls. "When suddenly, something took me back to where I'd come from, to the diaspora. I was still not really in my country. The young people didn't perceive me as one of them. And it hurt."

Someone else, at this point, might have broken, been overcome with self-pity. But Shaul turned the alienating attitude of his garin into a challenge.

MARCHING IN THE NETHERLANDS

Toward the end of basic training, they were offered a great opportunity.

The International Four Days March has taken place every year in the town of Nijmegen in the Netherlands , except during the two world wars. A competition, it is held between military and civilian groups from all over the world, who march for four consecutive days along a hilly course - in the Netherlands of all countries - which is mostly flat. The winner of the competition is the group that marches the fastest and most beautifully.

In order to choose the best team to send from Israel, the Israeli Defense Force held a competition within and between the different units. Every day, they walked 25 miles or ran about 15 with full gear. They had to reach the finish line within a certain time. For Shaul, this training course was another test, and he was determined to get through it and prove to his sabra friends that he was as good as they were. He didn't know how he would walk so far with his flat feet, but knew that he would, no matter what.

Training for the competition lasted three months, and every day, more and more soldiers dropped out. Shaul kept walking despite the burning pain in his feet, without saying a word. He walked as if his life depended on it, and every step he took made his body and mind stronger. To him, the walk represented a metamorphosis in which he changed from being a weak, delicate refugee in the eyes of the other soldiers into a strong man who could overcome any obstacle. During the entire training period, he was the only soldier who did

138

not miss a single day, and he was always one of the first to reach the finish line. Finally, a delegation to represent Nahal Hof, Shaul's battalion, was formed and Shaul and most of the boys in his garin were part of it. A competition was then held between the units, and in this competition, too, he did his part and stood out as a very dedicated and determined marcher.

The rules of the competition were brutal, because if any of the soldiers in the delegation broke, the whole group would be disqualified. If any of them showed signs of weakness, their teammates would immediately support him on both sides. In the end, the Nahal Hof team won and was chosen to represent the Israeli Defense Force (IDF).

This was followed by an order from Prime Minister Ben-Gurion: anyone representing the State of Israel has to immediately change his name if it is not Israeli. And so, Charlie David Hilsberg, who became Charles Van Bergen during the war and then Shaul Hilsberg when he immigrated to Israel, changed his name again, but for the last time, and became Shaul Harel.

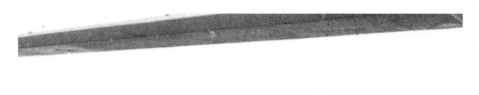

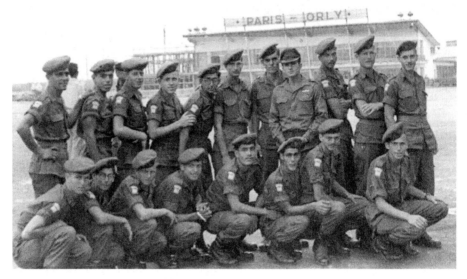

The delegation to the Four Days March at the airport in Paris—Shaul is in the
bottom row, fourth from the left

Because the Israeli delegation was expected to be hosted by the Jews of Nijmegen and other dignitaries, and since it was a group of Israelis who lacked
any manners and had never left the country, they were unaware of European
etiquette. The group was given a crash course in table manners from the high
priestess of proper conduct in society, none other than Hanna Bavly herself.

They learned things they had never known including: how to use cutlery
from the outside in and not the other way around, as they thought; how to eat
with their mouths closed; how to wipe their mouths with a napkin, and more.
However, Hanna Bavly forgot to teach them what the bowl of lemon juice was
for. They were served fish, and she hadn't explained that it was for washing
their hands at the end of the meal to get rid of the smell. When the soldiers

were invited to a fancy fish dinner with their hosts and saw the bowl with the lemon juice on the table, they drank it. The polite hosts were embarrassed and didn't know how to react, but as they didn't want to embarrass their amusing guests, they also drank the lemon juice, as if that was what it was there for.

Training in the Netherlands before the competition began. Shaul made an enormous effort there, too, greater than anyone else, and slowly became one of the leaders of the Israeli delegation. When the competition began, he and his friends supported anyone experiencing difficulty and led the Israeli team on a fast march. They were singing as they crossed the finish line and won.

By then, it was already clear that he had finally jumped over the tough Sabra hurdle. He was accepted by the group and became their friend.

When they returned triumphant from the competition, they were honored by the Chief of Staff, Moshe Dayan, with a visit to their base.

"Do you see this soldier?" The doctor who had accompanied them pointed at Shaul. "This soldier has flat feet, and anyone who examines him finds it hard to believe that he could have walked on them for so long, and still, he never missed a single day of training, which lasted three months!"

"Then I think we should remove the section about flat feet in profiles," said Moshe Dayan.

NOVEMBER 1956—THE SINAI CAMPAIGN: SORRY, LEAVE THE INJURED BEHIND

After returning to Israel after the march in the Netherlands and completing basic training, Shaul joined the Sollelim Garin, which was mixed. With this garin, he made it to the Nahal Paratroopers and began training. Israel was just eight years old, and despite the attacks by Palestinian fedayeen, there was an optimistic feel in the air.

However, the raids by the fedayeen increased, the Suez Canal was nationalized by Gamal Abdel Nasser, the president of Egypt, and Israel decided to cooperate with the British and French in an operation to capture Sinai and the Suez Canal.

Shaul and his comrades joined the Sinai Campaign in November 1956, before completing their paratrooper training. They were sent to a pick-up point in the south and were attached to the 51st Battalion of the Golani Brigade. Back then, the Golani Brigade didn't have the good reputation it has now, and the decision was to boost it with the help of Nahal spearhead units, which would serve as tank-carried infantry. They would be completely exposed on the turret. Today, that military concept is considered to be on the odd side and perhaps was taken from Russian warfare. For two weeks, the soldiers practiced climbing on and off the tanks, the plan being that the tanks would first run over the Egyptians, and then the Nahal soldiers would quickly jump off into the enemy trenches and finish the job.

Shaul, who was just 19, once again felt like he was facing the danger of death, but this time as an adult and with free will, a weapon and protection. Still, the danger to their lives was tangible and immediate.

The night before they left for the battlefield, Shaul wrote farewell letters to his relatives and wondered to himself if it was the last night of his life. Then he and his friends watched a French ship shelling the field to "soften it up" for them.

They climbed into half-tracks and drove down the sandy road leading to the outposts at Rafah Junction. Two half-tracks got stuck in the sand and couldn't move. The commander ordered the soldiers in the half-tracks to cram in with those who could. They were then delayed by the group that Shaul had to join, who had severe disciplinary issues and a few of the soldiers objected to having more soldiers with all their load bearing equipment crowd in with them. Shaul's spirits fell when he saw how his comrades were behaving. They were about to refuse the order, but then the platoon commander pulled out his pistol and shouted hoarsely that he would shoot anyone who didn't jump in. Having no choice, the reluctant soldiers climbed in and advanced toward their target, the Rafah outposts, where they were transferred onto tanks.

And then they were taken by surprise. They drove straight into a minefield and an Egyptian ambush, who must have received intelligence regarding the attack. The Egyptians lit up the field, painting the sky with artificial light and exposing them to a brutal barrage of fire. The two tanks in front of Shaul's were hit and caught fire, as did Shaul's and the tank that his good friend from Aloney Yitzchak, Arie Shtro was on.   From the blast, they flew a few feet through the air only to discover to their horror that they were in a minefield. They frantically started digging into the sand only to discover that they were in quicksand. They lay there helplessly, not knowing how to proceed.

Shaul believes that it was in those moments of terror that his hair started to turn white. The fear of death hung in the air and not all of the soldiers could take it. The three lying next to Shaul in the makeshift trench thought of making a run for it. "Let's get the hell out of here," one of them said.

Shaul was shocked by their cowardly and defeatist reaction and knew that if even one of them defied orders and ran off, the others would follow, and they would all be exposed to the mines, Egyptian fire and killed on the spot. And so, he immediately punched the soldier, glared at the other two and hissed loudly, "Shut up and keep fighting!"

They did as he said.

Their marvelous battalion commander Meir Pilewski, who later changed his name to Meir Pa'il, fearlessly and calmly led the impossible battle. In the end, with the help of the combat engineering corps, they courageously organized a new axis for the tanks to cross under the hellish fire, and before dawn, the Nahal soldiers and tanks returned and stormed the junction outposts

Shaul's platoon, Spearhead 1, was chosen to attack. They again climbed onto the tanks and advanced while firing constantly at the Egyptian positions. They were an easy target.

The Egyptians responded immediately and started firing back at them, and because they were sitting on the tanks and not inside them, it was easy to hit them. One soldier was wounded, followed by Shaul, who took a bullet in his left arm and a burst of fire in his groin. He immediately started to bleed heavily, and keeping his wits about him, he pressed his right hand on the wound in his arm and with his left, tried to stop the bleeding vein in his groin. The loss of blood made him faint, but he could still hear the following exchange over the two-way radio:

The tank commander shouted, "I have two seriously wounded. I need to stop to treat them."

The company commander responded, "Don't stop no matter what. If you have to, move on without the wounded."

Shaul couldn't believe what he was hearing, He was afraid that he'd die if he didn't receive immediate medical attention, but there was nothing he could do.

When the Israeli tanks arrived at the outpost and the soldiers jumped off into the trenches, the Egyptians ran off. Shaul and the other wounded man were rolled from the tank into the trench, and Shaul fell between the fleeing Egyptians.

He lay there for a long time, hanging between life and death, pressing as hard as he could on his injuries. The other wounded man was no longer breathing. He had no idea how long it took to take the outpost and before they started looking for the wounded. But he survived the severe injury, too.

As there were no rescue helicopters then, so he received only first aid. He was transferred by half-track to the collection point and from there in a van (there were no ambulances then either) from Rafah to Tel Hashomer Hospital. It was a long and painful trip.

The Sinai Campaign was a controversial operation. Some saw it as vital in light of the fedayeen attacks and the closure of the canal to Israel. Others saw it as a bitter mistake that placed Israel at the forefront of imperialist states such as France and England and wiped out any chance, however slim, to reach some sort of agreement with the Arab countries, first and foremost with Egypt.

It could have been ironic if Shaul, a Holocaust survivor, had lost his life when at only 19 in an operation whose contribution was controversial, cost 180 lives and earned Israel only three months of control of the Sinai Peninsula.

Saying that, the operation greatly reduced the number of fedayeen attacks (which some people claim were initiated by Nasser, who was already working up to the bigger conflict about ten years later). It brought about a period of relative calm that was the longest in the history of the State of Israel within the boundaries of the Green Line. Israel, which had barely recovered from the War of Independence, could therefore begin to evolve and carve its way.

NOVEMBER 1956–INJURED, HOSPITALIZED AND DECIDING TO BECOME A DOCTOR

Once he made it to Tel Hashomer Hospital, Shaul was operated on immediately and hospitalized for two months. Although his life had been saved, he had lost all sensation in his left hand. Worse than that, because his urethra had been injured, he was concerned that his sexual function and ability to have children would be permanently impaired. To a young man who dreamed of love and of starting a family, a Holocaust survivor who wanted continuity more than anything, it was like a death sentence.

But again, it turned out that his spirit could overcome any obstacle. His joy and gratitude for surviving, along with the supportive and supportive bond between the wounded, encouraged him. The humor in his ward was dark, and every time a girl came to visit the wounded, they would say, "Go sit with Shaul, with him there's no danger of anything happening to you..."

But fate shined on the young man who tried bravely to cope with his severe injury.

The nurses used to wash the soldiers every day. One day, when one of the nurses was washing Shaul, a "positive reaction" occurred.

The rumor spread and the hospital corridors were filled with cheers of joy and whistles of admiration: "He had an erection!" The news spread in whispers. The flagpole had been raised.

During the long weeks that he was bedridden, Shaul thought deeply about the almost supernatural impact that the doctor treating him had had on him, with the compassionate and intelligent look in his eyes, his white robe and soothing tone. Shaul knew that he could trust him.

He realized what a great privilege it was to work in such a profession, and he became inspired. He initially had been drawn to studying chemical engineering at the Technion, but he changed his mind. He would become a doctor. He would help save lives, heal people, alleviate or reduce their suffering, help them, and give back the thrill of life to those who had been broken. Suddenly, everything became clear: he had found his vocation and meaning in life.

In May 1957, Shaul was released from the army with a 35 percent disability and the honorable rank of private (later, as a doctor, he became a major).

He had served for only a year-and-a-half. He was also decorated by the commander of the 51st Battalion, Meir Pilevsky. The ceremony was not as grand as they are today. All he received was a page that read: "By your quiet demeanor and composure, you helped the battalion move quickly without being detained until the tanks could stop to take care of you."

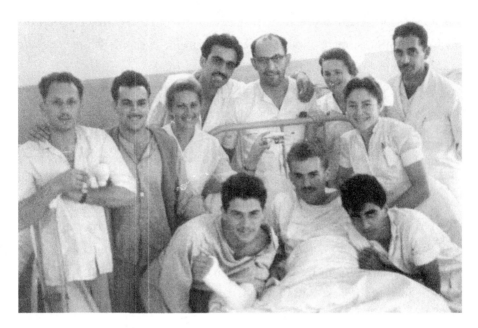

Shaul in a cast—first from the left in the first three

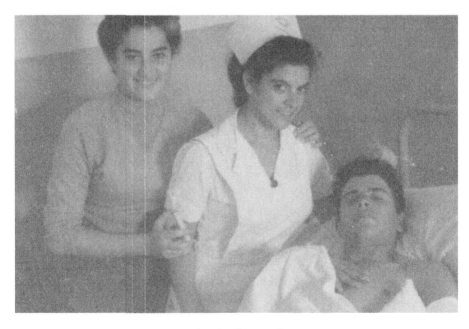

Shaul in hospital

1957—HAVING TEA WITH THE DOWAGER QUEEN OF BELGIUM AND THE BELGIAN CHIEF OF STAFF, AND AN UNFORGETTABLE ENCOUNTER

Romi Goldmuntz, the generous Zionist Belgian diamond dealer and patron saint of the Jewish Belgian children in Israel was celebrating his 75th birthday.

The Belgian government decided to surprise him and invite one of the hidden children he'd helped to the impressive party in his honor. Shaul Harel was chosen to represent the children.

The hidden boy, who had spent his childhood lacking love and food, entered the huge, glittering hall dressed in elegant tails and his eyes grew wide with astonishment. He stared at the heavy chandeliers hanging from the high ceiling, marveled at the honorable occasion and his eyes widened when he saw the Belgian women of nobility in their rustling dresses and dripping in gold, diamonds, emeralds and jade. His arm was still in a sling and he was wearing his war decoration from the Sinai Campaign, but he was wearing an elegant tuxedo and a bow tie.

Not far from him, the Dowager Queen Elisabeth was sitting drinking daintily from a gilded porcelain tea cup, her baby finger raised high. An impressive orchestra was playing dancing music, and Shaul found himself swept merrily away into the middle of the dance floor.

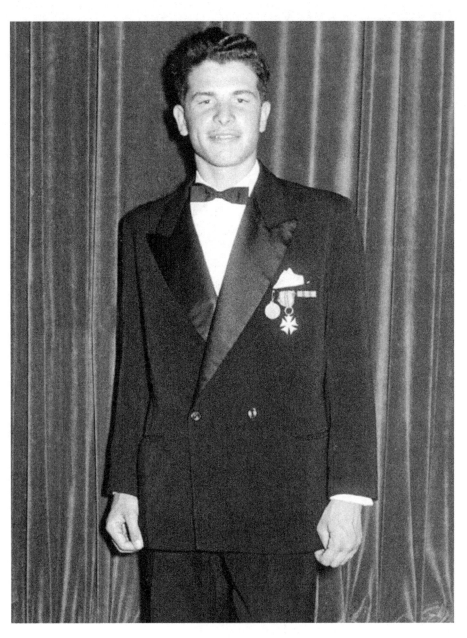

Shaul at the dance held by the Dowager Queen of Belgium

It became known that he was seriously wounded in the war and had even been decorated by the IDF for his bravery. He was seen as an Israeli war hero and given the honor of meeting the heads of state. The Belgian chief of staff started questioning him about the battles and strategy used during the war. It was hard for Shaul to be candid and speak about the horror he experienced and the chaos he witnessed in battle.

The next day, Shaul went out to a local bar in Brussels where he invited a nice young woman to dance. They began to speak in broken English but soon realized that they both spoke Hebrew.

"Where are you from," the young woman asked, "and what are you doing here?"

Shaul told her why he was there, that he'd been sent from Israel after being wounded in the Sinai War to participate in an event in honor of a man who has contributed greatly to Youth Aliya.

"Where were you injured?" the young woman interrupted him, her voice emotional.

"I fought in Rafah at the outposts and that's where I was wounded," he replied.

The woman started to tremor, and she started sobbing. Her slender body shook, and she would have collapsed if Shaul, surprised and embarrassed, hadn't taken her in his arms.

After she calmed down, he asked her why she'd reacted that way, and all color drained from his face when she did.

"My husband," she said, tears welling in her eyes again, "was an officer in the armored corps and he was killed at the junction." She told Shaul his name.

Shaul started trembling. As if in a nightmare, all the horrific images came rushing back...of those long moments after he was injured and of waiting for hours in the tank to be evacuated; of the officer, whom he now knew was the woman's husband, lying beside him dead and covered with a blanket.

Shaul couldn't stop trembling, and he will never forget how fate had brought him and the wife of his brother in arms together and how his friend had been killed, while he was rescued from that hellhole. He tossed and turned for nights, unable to sleep.

After the birthday party for Goldmuntz, Shaul was given 50 dollars a day for a month, so that he had some spending money for the trip. He saved a large portion of it and bought himself a Vespa with a flashlight on the wheel. At the time, it was one of the few in the Hebrew University's parking lot, and everybody assumed that he came from a wealthy family.

THE ROAD TO THE FACULTY OF MEDICINE

It was the end of the summer of 1957, and Shaul was now 20 years old. He didn't have a permanent home, no parents to guide him, and he had to pave his future path on his own. Both his brother and sister had families of their own to take care of. They each had a son and a daughter, and their financial situation wasn't good.

As he was released from the army in the middle of the academic year, he couldn't register yet for medical school, and he also knew how difficult it was to get in to the prestigious faculty. As such, he decided to register in the meanwhile to study physics and math, so that if he wasn't not accepted into medical school, he could at least get into chemical engineering, as he'd wanted to in his youth. Physics and math would give him a good basis for it.

He was happy to run into his former Nahal commander at the first lesson, Judd Ne'eman. Judd had been a tough commander, and during basic training, he forced Shaul to dig a three-by-three foot pit, only because he jumped over the fence to meet his girlfriend for a few minutes when he should have been with the battalion. That didn't stop the two young men from embracing happily or from developing a friendship that is still going strong.

Both Shaul and Judd immediately realized that math was not for them. There were a few geniuses in their class who would become very famous. They could solve problems in minutes, while all the other students watched in amazement and then copied their solutions. Shaul and Judd dropped out

153

of the math and physics courses.

One of Shaul's flat mates was a dentistry student by the name of Itzik Binderman. Shaul took a keen interest in the dentistry program and knew that as it was what he wanted and liked; he had to get into medical school.

He started auditing natural science lectures, keenly devouring every word of the lecturers.

Student life at that time was not easy. Shaul, like many others, shared a three-room apartment with eight other students. Their landlords, an elderly religious couple, lived in a small room in the middle of the apartment, from where they watched their comings and goings. The tenants were not allowed to bring girls home after 7:00 PM and the girls often had to sneak out through the window. To save on expenses, the boiler was turned on once a week. At one point, the landlord decided that they were using too much power to prepare dinner and suggested that he cook the eggs for them. One of the tenants came from a farming community and would bring them huge eggs. Somehow, tiny omelets resulted from those eggs, so small they could have been quail.

After discussing all the aspects of the situation, the resourceful students decided to write a name on every egg they gave to the landlord. The landlord would return the shell to the owner after cooking it, and thus they assured themselves a full portion of protein.

As most of the students had whole families to rely on, or at least some family, they had somewhere to go on the weekends. Every weekend, Shaul found himself with the problem of where to go. Not only his sibling's living conditions were an issue but his were as well. As an acclaimed bachelor, Shaul's waking hours didn't always suit his brother's family, and after losing the front door key once, he decided not to inconvenience them anymore.

And so, almost every weekend, Shaul found himself "homeless" and looking for a place to go with one of his friends. Sometimes he would spend the weekend with Shaul Yatziv from Aloney Yitzchak or Amir Makov from Rehovot, whom he met abroad and whose family was always welcoming.

Yitzchak Binderman, his flat mate, would also often invite him to stay with his hospitable and friendly family.

He was also always welcome to stay with his father's cousin Moteleh and his wife Hindeleh, who had a small apartment, but it seemed to have the magical ability of growing with the number of guests they had. Although Shaul would sometimes find himself staring into the eyes of a carp fish that he was sharing the bathroom with, he always felt at home there.

FALL 1958—FINALLY, A MEDICAL STUDENT

Although Shaul had attained his high school diploma, his results were far from great. But a man like Shaul wouldn't let facts keep him from his dream. He'd jumped over bigger hurdles in the past.

Getting into medical school has never been easy, although at the time, with all the new immigrants, the university was considerate of potential students with unimpressive high school diplomas and offered them the opportunity of taking two entrance exams. If they achieved particularly good results, they were given an interview. Still, there were only 51 spots, 24 of which were divided up as follows: Military students received 18, and Mizrachi students, women and Arabs got two spots each. The children of doctors, by the way, were given extra points! This meant that there were only 27 spots that Shaul could compete for.

And yet, against all odds, and even though their parents weren't doctors, and their matriculation scores were low, Shaul and his friend Shaul Yatziv from Aloney Yitzchak, managed to get in. He believed this was because of the excellent grades that he got in the entrance exams in chemistry and philosophy, after he worked hard, and thanks to the personal interview and admissions committee, whom he must have impressed.

Years later, when he was rummaging through his personal documents at Aloney Yitzchak, he found a moving letter of recommendation in regard to him and his friend, which Yehiel Harif had sent to the dean of the faculty of medicine, Prof. Privas.

This is what he wrote in October 1958.

> "As I know that you belong to the admissions committee, I am allowing myself to contact you and give you my opinion that both our boys deserve to be encouraged, both because of their ability to learn and because of their situation. They are Holocaust survivors who worked hard and were driven to attain a good education."

That's when Shaul realized to what extent their beloved principal had contributed to shaping their lives.

1958-1963—HAVING FUN WHILE MAKING A LIVING

After being accepted into medical school, Shaul moved with Shaul Yatziv to the student dorms in Givat Ram, in Jerusalem. It was a lively place, and the students would meet every evening in the dining room. They cooked for themselves and organized a dancing party every week. The two Shauls soon stood out as excellent dancers, and Shaul Harel was crowned once a champion of the Twist.

Shaul had to deal with financing his studies and upkeep throughout his time at university. "Luckily," as he had been wounded in the war and the IDF agreed to grant him a one-time student loan, but he still had to find work, and quick.

Shaul was a diligent student but he worked, too. He had to work in a variety of casual jobs, and he used all of his skills—even those he didn't have—in order to convince employers to hire him.

He taught ping pong at the university, worked as a construction worker for the university when the Givat Ram campus was being built, he was an assistant to a gardener, an usher at YMCA concerts, and as part of a project to help new immigrants to learn Hebrew, he went twice a week to Mevaseret Zion to read the newspaper to immigrants from Cochi.

After a while, he decided he needed to improve his earning capacity, and started using his innovation and production instincts, along with his business sense. He joined forces with a young photographer after suggesting a deal.

The idea was simple but was based on a deep understanding of "Polish" psychology: they knocked on people's doors and offered to take pictures of their children for free, with no obligation to buy the pictures: "If you want to buy it when you see it, you can, but you don't have to."

Shaul and his friend went home, developed the photos and returned with the developed photos. "Look how beautiful your child looks here," Shaul would say as he gave the embarrassed yet proud mothers one of his captivating smiles.

"Yes," the mother would agree. "He really is a beautiful child. How much would you like for the picture?"

Despite his money problems, he enjoyed life to the fullest, and after visiting European countries at the end of 1957 as an emissary for Youth Aliya, he again had the urge to travel. And so, after his first year of medical school, in the summer of '59, he went off on his first trip alone with a little bit of money, a backpack, and naturally, an Israeli flag. In those days, Israel was still very popular, and the flag could help to hitch rides. He met Amir Makov, a student from the Technion, on the flight from Tel Aviv to Athens. He was also on his way to Europe. They clicked immediately and became life-long friends.

They had a wonderful trip, full of adventures and new experiences. They hitchhiked through some countries, proudly waving the Israeli flag. In others, they rented a car, and that was basically when Shaul learned how to drive.

One experience, in Newcastle, the gloomy northern capital of England, made a deep impression on them. They arrived in the dismal and rainy city in the evening and started searching in vain for a place to stay. Their biggest disappointment was when the sexton of the city's synagogue refused to help them.

Having no choice, they went to the Salvation Army, assuming that it was a kind of military boarding school (army, right?). They had no idea that it was a place of refuge for all the down and out of Newcastle. It was dark by the time they got to the dreary gray building, and they had no choice but to accept what they were offered, each on a different floor: a tiny nook with a bed and bedding that hadn't been changed in eons, if their color and stains were anything to go by. When they complained about the filthy bedding, the gatekeeper gave them a piece of his mind: "You and your demands! Just be grateful that two occupants died yesterday, and that's why we have room for you."

They lay fully dressed and shivering all night long, afraid to close their eyes and every now and then, pushing away mysterious hands invading their space and trying to steal their luggage.

In the morning, happy to be alive, they were served thin porridge with all the needy people, and then ran away and decided to find a better solution. Being resourceful Israelis, they went to the synagogue again and enthusiastically told the sexton how well the Anglican Church had taken care of them and found them a place to sleep in a spacious home in the city. Naturally, the sexton felt uncomfortable hearing how welcoming the gentiles had been, and the problem of a place to stay for the following nights was solved.

Amir and Shaul have never forgotten that trip and they have remained fast friends ever since. Amir, who comes from a well-known and established family from Rehovot would often invite Shaul to stay for the weekend, and Shaul truly enjoyed the heartfelt welcome he received from them all.

In the summer of 1960, Shaul came across an ad for a great job that read: We are looking for talented, French-speaking entertainers for an interesting position with the Jewish Agency called "Getting to Know Israel." It was signed by Puts'u (the author and poet Israel Weisler).

The job involved traveling to Europe on the dilapidated boat Artsa, which was previously used as an illegal immigrant boat. It was to serve as a floating youth hostel. The aim was to collect young Belgians, Italians, French and Swiss between the ages of 16 and 22 and to bring them to Israel. They would have entertainment in the evenings, during which they would play social games and learn a little Hebrew, a little Zionist history and Israeli songs and dances. Then, after arriving in Israel, they would take them on trips around the country, stay on a kibbutz, and then after three weeks, take them back to their countries, hopefully with a warm place for Israel in their hearts.

Shaul imagined how he would take a bunch of beautiful European girls on his Vespa to show them how wonderful Israel was, and how wonderful he himself was. He was also excited at the possibility of continuing to travel through Europe and to visit ports such as Genoa, Naples, Marseille.

Highly motivated, Shaul asked for an interview.

"What can you do?" Puts'u asked, his enormous mustache rising and falling like sails in the wind. The student Shaul, who saw the hidden potential of this job, kept his head. "I speak French and I can teach folk dancing and organize social activities."

The mustache smiled, nodded and hired him on the spot

Once on board, Shaul met the rest of the entertainment crew, but he was the only one who spoke fluent French. All the others had bluffed their way in.

The downside of the job was the bad condition of the boat. It was old and neglected and could barely carry a hundred passengers. That didn't stop them from cramming on 250 each time. It was so overcrowded that not everyone had a place to sleep.

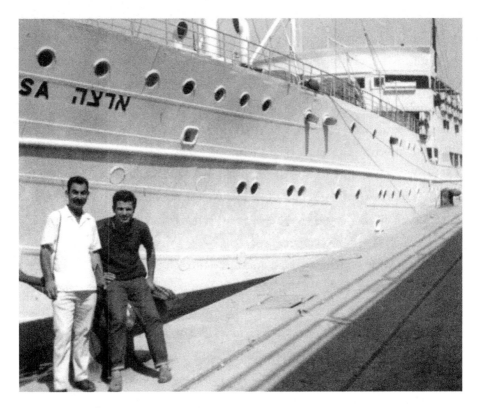

Shaul with Puts'u next to the Artsa

Naturally, it was humid and there was no air conditioning, the deck was packed and some of the passengers had to sleep in the lifeboats. All of them were young and clearly, their hormones were raging, as were those of the crew.

Since it was his job to organize social activities for the young visitors, he started decorating and setting up the small lobby, which included a bar. It was the only place where they could gather for social activities, sing and dance. Shaul found out that the sailors were partners in the bar, and one of them, who was rude and conniving, had taken over. He was smuggling liquor and wanting to make a profit selling it to the young passengers. He didn't like the fact that Shaul had "robbed him" of them for cultural purposes and was preventing him from making a buck off the passengers. Mostly, he disliked the fact that Shaul didn't back off, panic or give in to his demands.

The sailor said to Shaul, "Go away, and take your idiotic games with you."

But Shaul simply looked at the brute and responded coolly, "I'm sorry, but it's my job to provide them with social activities."

"Oh, is that right?" the sailor said meanly. "Then I'll see you at the stern." To make his point, he popped one of the balloons that Shaul had hung in the lobby with his cigarette.

Shaul immediately went to find out what it meant to meet at the stern.

Much to his unease, he was told that it was where the sailors would take revenge against anyone they didn't like. For example, customs officers would sometimes plant snitches who would report smugglers to them.

When the smugglers happened to catch a snitch, they would throw all of his belongings overboard, including his glasses if he had any, and then take him to the stern, wrap his head and body in a large sack, beat the hell out of him, and threaten to throw the sack into the sea.

With all due respect to his courage, Shaul didn't want a violent struggle with the rowdy sailors, who may put him in mortal danger.

Luckily, he'd become good friends with the boatswain, who happened to be a big strong man and liked him. When Shaul told him about his run-in with the sailor and the threats he had made, the captain reassured him in his deep voice: "Shaul, my friend, don't give it a moment's thought. As long as I'm on this ship, no one will touch even a hair on your head."

And Shaul's hair was indeed never harmed, as the boatswain summoned the violent sailor to "talk" and quietly explained to him why it was worth his while to leave Shaul alone.

But that was not the end of Shaul's adventures on the Zionist "Love Boat."

On each voyage, as he'd hoped when he signed up to work on the boat, he found a nice girl to take on trips around Israel. He was highly successful (Puts'u would someday claim that Shaul left him only crumbs).

163

It was six o'clock when Shaul's Vespa sliced through the air and came to a screeching stop on the pier. And at precisely six o'clock, the boat was supposed to leave the pier and set sail. To Shaul's dismay, he watched as the bow of the boat began to slowly move away.

"Are you crazy?" Puts'u thundered angrily at Shaul. "Where were you? What happened? And what will we do now? What about the French?"

Shaul was looking at the police barricade preventing him from going in when he heard another shout: "Quick, jump now!"

A sailor at the bow of the ship threw Shaul a rope. Within tenths of a second, he estimated the distance of the boat from the shore and without thinking twice, he jumped, caught the rope and was pulled onboard.

The applause and whistles of admiration didn't last long. The captain summoned Shaul to his room, put him on trial and fined him.

The report noted:

> "Entertainer Harel has been fined the sum of ten Israeli pounds for not reporting on board after shore leave and for jumping from the pier to the boat while it was already maneuvering its way out to sea."

s. s. ARTSA ארצה אׁק

<u>Extract from Official Log Book Voy 207</u>

July the 18th at 1955 hrs
Haifa

Entertainer Israel Shaul Seaman's book 4616
has been fined the sum of Il 10.00 (Ten Israel
Pounds) for not reporting on board at the
termination of shore leave and for jumping
from quay to ship while ship was allready
manoeuvering on it's way out of port.

....
Chief Officer

....
Master

6/52 G. 60 150·100 נוי

The fine Shaul was given

165

Shaul was very proud of this document and has always displayed it in a place of honor on the wall of his office, next to his professional certificates.

Shaul made new friends that summer. One of them was Philippe Lambert from France, who was only 17 in the summer of 1960. Philippe was sent by his parents on the *Artsa* to visit Israel with a French youth group.

Two years later, Shaul went on a student exchange trip with Judd Ne'eman. Naturally, they didn't miss the opportunity of taking a road trip to the south of France first. They rented a Citroën 2CV, or *deux chevaux*, as the locals called it. It was a popular car in France at the time, and its great advantage was that you could take out the seats and sleep in it. It was also the quickest way to meet girls at the bar or on the beach, and a sure-fire way to attract them.

Sometimes, if they met a girl who one of them liked, they would argue whether to stay another day in the town or move on. Usually, they reached a compromise.

On their way south, they went to visit Philippe in Macon. His parents wanted to thank Shaul for being so kind to their son when he was visiting Israel and decided to spoil their young Israeli guests. They did so by taking them to the most expensive and well-known restaurant in the area, 12 miles away.

It was only when they got there that they discovered, much to Judd's dismay, that the restaurant specialized only in snails. "I couldn't possibly eat those things," he whispered in horror to Shaul, who was looking at his plate with utter pleasure. "They disgust me. As soon as a snail's head enters my body, I'll puke, and that'll be very unpleasant."

So as not to offend their generous hosts, they told them that Judd was really, really allergic to snails, and that he could die if he took even one bite. Judd ended up eating an omelet, the plainest and most basic food ever served at the highly regarded restaurant.

That year, when Shaul and Judd returned to Paris after a trip around France, they joined a student exchange program and started working at a hospital.

They both loved Paris, but Judd had become enraptured with the magic of cinema (this was during the French New Wave). When it came time to return to Israel, Judd decided in the spur of the moment to drop out of medical school and stay in Europe.

Shaul returned to Israel alone. When the academic year began, he had a difficult time coming up with excuses for Judd's absence. He rushed off letters to France and urged Judd to come back. "It's a shame. Medicine can give you a great economic foundation and then you can also become a director. After all, you can combine your art with medicine."

Shaul didn't let up and eventually Judd returned to Israel, caught up and became a doctor.

Between shifts in the emergency room, Judd began to make movies and became one of the top cinematography lecturers at Tel Aviv University. In fact, he received the title of professor (of cinema) even before Shaul and won the Israel Prize for Cinema.

Between one job and another, and his wild student life, Shaul managed to complete his medical degree. It wasn't easy in the beginning. When the students stood facing their first human body and learned about the internal organs, many of them felt sick to the stomach but they slowly got used to it and eventually it got to a point where, without thinking anything of it, they'd take their sandwiches out of their bags and eat it right over a body. Some of them even fell in love during the lessons and would hold hands over the body.

During his years at medical school, Shaul made some lifelong friendships, including with couples who were already married.

Shaul became one of the last bachelors in his year, although he was not even 26 years old. Yes, people married young then. But Shaul had not had a long relationship since his first girlfriend at Aloney Yitzchak. He was known as a charming Don Juan whose intentions were not serious. He was friends with Shuka and Ahuva Iron, who he would visit occasionally for a meal, with Yehuda Shapira and his wife Naomi, who lived in the Jerusalem Talpiot neighborhood, on the border close to the Jordanian border posts, and he would get there on his Vespa, his heart racing a little faster. The homes of his married friends would also serve as a refuge for him on weekends, when everyone went away, and the student dorms emptied out.

And of course, there was Judd, his tough commander from the army who had become his closest friend. They studied together for exams, traveled around Israel together, and as mentioned, abroad. Shaul would drive Judd around on his Vespa. One day they tried to buy a car from the 1930s for 300 liras, a Ford that fell apart the first time they drove it up Shlomzion Street—the bottom of the car broke, and the breaks didn't work. They barely managed to jump out to save their lives after turning the car toward the curb. This left them with no choice but to stick with Shaul's Vespa, which they both remember as a slightly traumatic but amusing experience. Judd had long legs, a little too long in relation to Shaul's low Vespa. One day, when Shaul stopped at a red light, Judd relaxed and put his feet down on the road. When the light turned green and Shaul started moving, Judd found himself standing in his place. Shaul kept driving and talking enthusiastically to Judd behind him. The other drivers on the road, who saw the unusual spectacle of a man driving a Vespa and talking to himself (remember, there were no mobile phones or earbuds then), must have thought him insane and grasped their heads in anger.

Shaul and Philippe lost contact until 40 years later, when Shaul received a phone call from a man who had just returned from a trip to France.

The man had called to give him Philippe's regards and told him that on his last trip, he visited a small town near Avignon surrounded by vineyards. He stayed at a B&B in a magnificent old building that was once the residence of a bishop, and when the proprietor found out that his guest was from Israel, he told him that he had a friend in Israel, Shaul Harel, who had been a medical student 40 years ago.

Delighted, Philippe asked him to look Shaul up and pass on his phone number. The man did all he could and found Shaul in the Medical Association's listing. Shaul was very moved, and although it had been 40 years since they'd last been in contact, they both felt as if it had been only yesterday.

Not long after, Shaul and his family visited Phillipe and his wife Elizabeth in their house near Avinion and they picked up where they'd left off.

STARTING A FAMILY AND SPECIALIZING IN MEDICINE

1940—HE'S IN BRUSSELS, SHE'S IN TEL AVIV

It was 1940, a few months after World War II broke out, and Shaul was still safe in the loving fold and home of his parents and siblings. At the end of February that year, a dramatic and significant event occurred that would change Shaul's life: Dalia, a sweet and beautiful baby girl with bright and curious eyes, came into the world and would one day be his wife and the mother of his children.

Dalia's mother Yehudit, and her father Israel, were born in the same small town of Budaniv in Galicia. It was near Ternopil and about 125 miles from Lviv. Lviv was once a wonderful, elegant city, the capital of Galicia and was under Austro-Hungarian rule until World War I when it fell under Polish Rule until it became part of Ukraine after World War II.

Israel came from a family in the horse-trading business and was considered a prodigy by the family. Yehudit lost her father when she was four years old and she and her brother helped her mother to run the simple workers' restaurant in town, which is where she learned to cook.

They were both active in the Gordonia youth movement and lived for a few years in Lviv before immigrating to Palestine.

There, Israel graduated from the Jewish Teachers Seminary, and Yehudit worked for a notary as a clerk (something she's always been proud of).

During these years, they also studied Hebrew, probably due to Israel's studies at the seminary and their activities in Gordonia.

After Yehudit's mother died, they received a fictitious marriage certificate and immigrated to Palestine in 1935. A few months later, they were married in a modest ceremony.

She was 24 and he was 26. They were the lucky ones, as both their large families had stayed in Galicia and were wiped out, except for two of Israel's nephews and one of Yehudit's nieces.

The economic situation in Palestine was bad and Yehudit had to work as a waitress, a job that she surprisingly stayed in until she was quite old. She enjoyed it because the artists and leaders of the community hung out in the Tel Aviv cafes, and she got to meet them.

Only after five years of marriage did the couple allow themselves to bring a child into the world, and never imagined that World War II would break out in the meanwhile, before Dalia was born. The first five months after the war broke out passed relatively peacefully. It was before the Germans occupied Belgium and the Hilsberg family began its exodus to France.

In May 1940, everything changed, and not only in Europe. The small Jewish community in Palestine started to become increasingly concerned, especially after the Italians based in Rhodes shelled Tel Aviv on September 9, 1940. It was the deadliest bombardment that Tel Aviv had ever known, and 117 of the city's residents and seven from the nearby Arab village of Summayl (now in the center of Tel Aviv) were killed, while 263 were wounded.

What's amazing is that the only thing that Yehudit ever mentioned of that traumatic event was how the people in the bomb shelter admired her gorgeous baby. Unlike many other residents of Tel Aviv who fled to Jerusalem, she and Israel decided to stay in Tel Aviv, which had become a ghost town overnight. Other than that incident, the war years passed relatively peacefully for little Dalia, but for her parents and the entire community, the future was more frightening. They lived in fear of an invasion by General Rommel, whose troops were positioned in North Africa. At one point, the leaders of the

Yishuv[2] even came up with a plan to prepare a last stand on Mount Carmel, kind of like the Maccabean on Mount Masada.

In the spring of 1945, when Charlie was almost eight and had already spent years in orphanages repressing all his experiences from the war, Dalia, an only child, was just starting to gather and retain every experience she had, even those of her close ones. She kept these safe in her heart and to this day, remembers every detail and date. At just over five years old, she would listen intently to the stories of the refugees who came to tell her parents what had happened to their families, almost all of whom had perished somewhere in Galicia. She absorbed the atmosphere of mourning in their home. Later, she would define her parents, who had lost almost all their family in Poland, as first-generation Holocaust survivors, and herself as second-generation.

Yehudit made sure that Dalia ate everything on her plate. Even during the 1950s, the period of austerity, Yehudit ran from farm to farm to find a little chicken and butter for her daughter. She would even try to stash a chicken under the bus seat, despite the risk of a confrontation with the tough inspectors.

Israel was a wise man, and he took care of Dalia's intellectual and spiritual nourishment—every day, he would bring home two books from the library for his bookworm of a daughter to satiate her lust for knowledge. She would devour them in no time, even when they were too advanced for her age, as the grave librarian explained.

Dalia's parents sent her to school when she was five-and-a-half. Lessons were held in the afternoon, as there was no room in the morning. They wasted no time.

They lived from hand-to-mouth, and Dalia had to share a room with her parents until she was eight as they shared an apartment with another family,

---

2   The Jewish population living in Palestine was called the Yishuv until the State of Israel was established in 1948.

like many of her friends. Still, Dalia grew up with the most important feeling of all: that she was loved by her parents.

Dalia would later pass on that love to her husband, and to her children too, of course. She would take care of Shaul with the devotion of a protective mother, as if to compensate him for his years without love, concern or pampering.

Dalia, born in the sand dunes of Tel Aviv, was a true Sabra in every aspect of her life, and a Zionist in her soul. She was rebellious and opinionated, and socially and politically involved even before she knew the meaning of those words.

She would chase after the British soldiers with a bunch of other kids her age while singing the song "Kalaniot[3]" to them. In the curfew of Operation Agatha, or Black Sabbath as it is sometimes called, when the British soldiers raided almost every home in search of weapons and making arrests, she went out onto the porch and noticed a British soldier watching her from the roof. Without hesitation and to her mother's horror, she spat angrily on the porch floor to express her contempt. The soldier watched her in amazement while her mother almost fainted.

When she was only in second grade, she wrote a letter to her friend, who was in the hospital. The literary influences in the flowery language she used was clear: "Today they hoisted our boys up on the gallows (Dov Gruner and his friend). God will avenge their blood."

Her friend gave her the letter years later when they were in high school.

Dalia had clear memories of things that happened when she was five, unlike Shaul, who repressed his memories from about the same age.

Whenever she is hit by a wave of despair regarding the current situation in Israel, she tries to go back to the beginning to cheer herself up...to the

---

3   The song was used as a code during the British Mandate to alert fighters of the Lehi and Etzel to the presence of British soldiers (their caps were of the color of the flower).

night that she heard that the Partition Plan had passed the UN vote and the indescribable buzz of excitement they all felt that day when she was eight. They all danced in circles in Dizengoff Square after Ben-Gurion announced the establishment of the State of Israel. She always says how lucky she was to be around for the most important milestones in Israel's history, both the good and the bad.

During the War of Independence, she had to stop learning and go from one bomb shelter to another. They didn't have one in their apartment building. The droning sound of Egyptian planes approaching and the deafening shelling of Tel Aviv in contrast with the utter silence in the shelter would haunt her for many nights to come. She remembers that when the *Altalena* (a ship bearing arms and recruits for Israel's War of Independence) reached the shores of Tel Aviv carrying weapons for the Irgun[4], the teachers ordered all the third graders to go to the teacher's room and lie quietly under the tables. But since they had no idea why, she lay there peacefully reading *Tarzan of the Apes* with one of the boys.

She remembers walking east with her parents and masses of people from Tel Aviv to get away from the shore and from the ship, which they were afraid would explode after it caught fire from the warning shots that the IDF fired. She remembers Menachem Begin's emotional speech and wondering how a grown man could be crying.

She remembers the period after the War of Independence, when she attended Tel Nordau and Hakalir Elementary Schools, and then Ironi Hey High School as a happy one. She was active in the elitist youth movement Mahanot Haolim (and tried in vain to figure out why the kibbutz movement split so dramatically into Ihud and Meuhad). The boys and girls her age felt safe, independent and free to go wherever they pleased. This, despite the fedayeen attacks, reprisal operations, skirmishes and Sinai Campaign. Was it because of

---

4   A Jewish military organization prior to 1948, in the Mandate Palestine period.

the euphoria that came with the first decade of Israeli independence?

As she finished school young, she was drafted into the Israeli Air Force a few months after she turned 17 but found herself extremely disappointed.

Not like today, the girls were given only dull jobs, which usually involved making coffee for the commanders, filling out lists of spare parts or typing the seminar papers for officers who were studying. Her mother urged her to take evening classes at the university during and after her military service, which she did for two years. She then decided to continue her studies at the Hebrew University.

Despite her inclination to the humanities, and taking future jobs opportunities into consideration, she took classes in economics and sociology.

Her living conditions in Jerusalem were quite modest. For the first year, she shared a room with a friend, and two guys lived in the other room. She wasn't used to the cold of Jerusalem, and as there was no central heating, they warmed up by a smoking kerosene heater. They would place orange peels on it to perfume the air. After finding it incredibly difficult to drag herself out from under her thick Polish duvet that her mother "shlepped" for her on the bus from Tel Aviv, she decided to spend all day in the warm hall of the Kaplan building.

Naturally, she soon became known as a very hard-working student. In her second year, she moved into an apartment with central heating but again shared a room with a friend. Later, she had her own room, but she always shared an apartment. At one point, there were five girls sharing one bustling apartment, with boys coming and going. In order to find work as soon as she completed her studies, she decided, despite her natural inclinations, to look for a job as an economist. Back then it was the profession of the future and an extremely popular degree to pursue. All the members of the socialist youth movements were suddenly charmed by the principles of the competitive capitalist world as presented to them by Prof. Dan Patinkin. Prof. Patinkin was of the American Chicago School neoclassical economic "school of thought," and his students learned that maximizing profit was of utmost importance. Later, as is well known, they tried furiously to apply it. Dalia, with her socialist and sociology background studying human behavior patterns, didn't agree.

In the first chapter of her career, between 1960 and 1969, she worked for the Ministry of Trade and Industry in the Mamilla building in Jerusalem, which is now the Waldorf Astoria Hotel. Jerusalem was then a quiet city, marvelously green, and had a splendor that Tel Aviv lacked. It was also divided. More than once, she took a wrong turn on her way to the office and was met with an amused glance from a Jordanian soldier looking at her over the wall, but she felt no tension.

Then she met Shaul.

AND THERE WAS DALIA, IN HER PAJAMAS

As a child, fate may have been against him, but it certainly made up for it later with love and marriage.

Dalia was a tall, attractive and intelligent young woman (too tall for her generation and taste), and she appeared in Shaul's life one evening in March 1963.

It was the eve of Purim, and Dalia's good friend and flat mate, Nili Keinan, may her memory be a blessing, invited her to a pajama party that the medical students were throwing. Nili told her that she'd met two young men abroad (remember the trip of 1959?): Amir Makov, who was an intellectual with incredible knowledge; and Shaul Harel, a medical student who was known for his zest for life. Shaul had asked her to bring a friend to the party for his friend from Aloney Yitzchak but forgot to mention the matter of height. His friend came up to Dalia's shoulder.

Shaul took one glance at the girl in fancy Chinese silk pajamas and took it all in: her beautiful face, her wise eyes, her long, shapely body…and that something inside that cannot be explained in words or with logical or neurological formulas…that mysterious element that made his heart race.

As it turned out, he'd already noticed her at the canteen in the Kaplan building at the Givat Ram campus, and mistakenly interpreted her natural shyness as arrogance and snobbery. And so, when she didn't respond immediately to his flirtations, he moved on to other girls and left the party without walking

Dalia home. This deeply annoyed her.

The next time they met, when Shaul came to visit Nili, he was met with a sour and angry face and realized that he didn't stand a chance.

But one evening, when he was going through a dry patch with the girls, he plucked up the courage to call her. To his surprise, she agreed to go on a date with him. Happily whistling one of his favorite tunes, he rode off on his Vespa, only to have it break down. It took him an hour-and-a-half to repair it.

Dalia simply forgave him for being late, that time and all the times that followed (after all, they didn't have phones at home), and they haven't parted since.

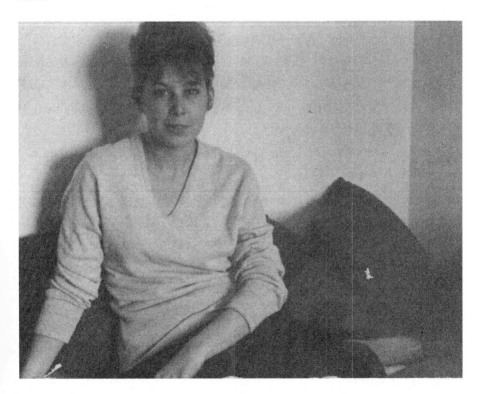

Dalia

DECEMBER 1963—I TAKE YOU TO BE MY WIFE AND "BUT DALIA, HE'S A REFUGEE"

Shaul found himself falling for Dalia. He had a feeling that they'd make a great team and willingly gave up his wild bachelor life. It took him only five months to know for sure that he'd found the one.

Shaul soon discovered Yehudit's fine cooking and may have made his decision to join the family because of her wonderful Galician-style gefilte fish, which was sweet, salty and peppery.

He wasn't overly romantic when he proposed, but he was very original and down to earth.

Instead of being kitsch and going down on one knee with a sparkling engagement ring in his hand and the lights of Paris or the Caribbean Islands in the background, as people do these days, Shaul's proposal was restrained, and in that lay its thrill:

"A three-room apartment on 21 Washington has come on the market," Shaul began. "I'll have my own room, and Judd will have his, and another guy, Amiram Hirschfeld, will take the third. How about moving in with me and saving on rent?"

Astonished, Dalia replied, "But Shaul, you know I can't do that, it's just not done."

To which Shaul replied, "Oh, clearly, we'll get married first, okay?"

Dalia's family still had barely a penny to their name and her parents were still living in the apartment where she was born, although they now had rights to the entire apartment. Her mother Yehudit was still working hard as a waitress (which Dalia didn't really like), but her father, despite being very smart, couldn't find permanent employment, which left her mother as the main breadwinner.

Dalia's mother was stunned because she barely knew Shaul. Still, she paid for the wedding and also for the two wedding rings they bought—one for Dalia, and one for Shaul.

They both thought that they read each other's character wrong. Shaul thought that he was marrying a very obliging, passive and attentive woman who would pamper him. Although he didn't lack any pampering, after the wedding he soon discovered that she had strong opinions and was at times rebellious. On her part, Dalia thought she'd caught a happy-go-lucky husband whose main interest was traveling and having fun, which would counter her own seriousness; that he wouldn't go further than being a health care fund doctor. But what did his career matter, when the main thing was to be happy? She didn't know that a highly ambitious and motivated man had come into her life and that he was planning to climb to the top.

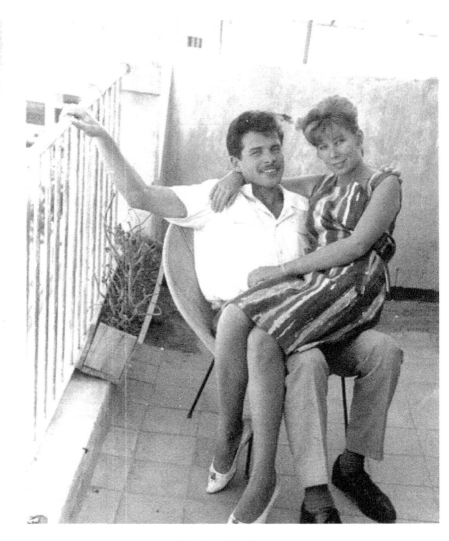

Shaul and Dalia

When she told a friend of hers who knew Shaul from the army that she was marrying him, she briefly got to feel as Shaul had as a refugee encountering Israeli sabras. He looked at her in pity and said, "But Dalia, he's a refugee."

Dalia got mad and retorted, "Yes, but he certainly looks more Israeli than you! In comparison, you look like you just stepped off the boat!"

The ceremony was held in December 1963, in the reception hall of a small synagogue on Geula Street in Tel Aviv, which had been leased to the Committee for the Wellbeing of Israel's Soldiers. Since Shaul was a disabled IDF veteran, he could have his wedding there for free. The meal was the usual main course of chicken thigh, mashed potatoes, peas and carrots, but the music—the music was special at the time, because they had a live band that Yehudit, Dalia's mother knew from work, and the atmosphere was great.

The newlyweds celebrated their honeymoon in Eilat at a motel, after a two-and-a- half-hour flight down on a Dakota. Eilat still looked like a desert town in the Wild West, and had only one fairly good restaurant. The weather was unusual for Eilat and it was cold and rainy and the motel provided no extra blankets, so they had to cover themselves with towels. The hotel manager raised an eyebrow—a honeymoon couple who needed more blankets? They couldn't change their flight back to Tel Aviv because there was only one flight a week.

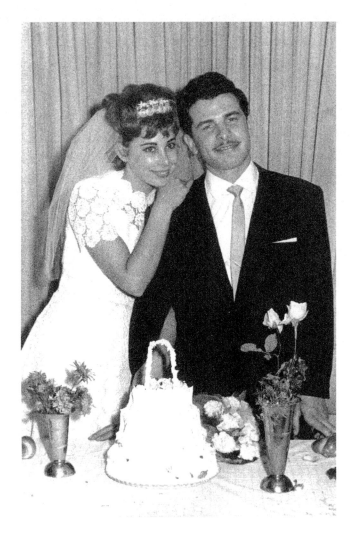

Shaul and Dalia on their wedding day

At the ripe old age of 26, as one of the last bachelors in his year, which in today's terms is very young, Shaul finally had a warm and stable home after moving from place to place practically all of his life until he got married. Yehudit welcomed him warmly into the family and he became like a son to her.

The wedding and honeymoon over, they returned to 21 Washington Street in Jerusalem. Shaul was in his last year of medical school and Dalia was working full-time at the Ministry of Industry and Trade and supported him.

It didn't take her long to realize that she had entered into marriage with another two men. Shaul felt bad about dining alone with her in the kitchen, and she would make dinner for the four of them. Naturally, none of the men could be trusted to clean their rooms, and so she found herself cleaning the whole apartment.

The apartment at 21 Washington Street didn't become famous for its interesting tenants, but rather because of the wild spontaneous parties that they threw. Shaul and Judd had a fixed and simple strategy: they would take buckets to the Mahane Yehuda market, fill them with hummus and tahini, pick up some pitas and pickles, add some semi dry red wine (very good, Adom Atik[5]), which they would sometimes mix with cheap vodka to get everyone drunk (including themselves). The rumor would spread around Jerusalem like wildfire, and dozens of youngsters would show up, turn up the music and dance until dawn.

---

5   Well into the 1980s, international wine books would still refer to Adom Atik when writing about Israel. It was the biggest selling table wine in export markets, sometimes exporting surprising quantities to the non-kosher market, in particular to Sweden. It is still sold today, although a bottle now costs a few dollars.

1965—INTERNSHIP AT ICHILOV HOSPITAL AND PROF. MARCUS

Upon graduation, when Shaul had to choose where to do his internship, there weren't many options. It's hard to believe, but back then, the Beilinson, Tel Hashomer and Ichilov hospitals weren't considered good internship options. They were seen as an academic wasteland, and all the students wanted to be in one place: Hadassah Hospital.

Shaul and Judd gave it a lot of thought, weighed the pros and cons, and managed to convince 15 interns, including Shaul's good friend Shuka Iron to go to Ichilov, of all places. As they saw it, there were plenty of good doctors at Hadassah Jerusalem, and the interns there were just that—interns. Ichilov, on the other hand, had a shortage of doctors. In addition, they knew their self-important professors from Hadassah, who ran a rigid hierarchy, were pompous and sometimes downright nasty. To them, the interns would always remain students.

This decision would turn out to be an extremely wise one because they got to work as doctors from the moment they started and gained hands-on experience. In fact, at a certain point, Shaul and his friends would work on their own in the emergency room, and they would get the doctor on duty only in severe cases. This gave them plenty of experience.

There were, of course, the groundbreakers of the generation under whom the interns worked: Prof. Dreyfus, the Head of the Internal Medicine

Department; Prof. Marcus, the Head of the Surgical Department; and Prof. Boger, the Head of Pediatrics. They were also multicultural and integrated general knowledge in their practice of medicine.

Prof. Marcus was a well-known surgeon and held in high esteem. He was an unusual but awe-inspiring man and had already been a great surgeon back in Germany before becoming one of the top surgeons in Israel. He worked mainly at Hadassah Tel Aviv Hospital, and then at Ichilov.

When the interns did the rounds with him, he would explain the cases to them while lecturing them on history, art and politics. When they stood around the operating table and saw him in action, they immediately realized that he was one of the best. He was strict and extroverted by nature, and no one dared to challenge his diagnoses.

When performing surgery, he would have one team of nurses in the operating room and another standing by to replace them. If he asked a nurse for seven inches of thread and she handed him eight, he would stop for a moment and sullenly order, "Get me a different nurse!" and the poor woman would be sent packing while another, quivering nurse from the backup team would replace her. Sometimes, one of the senior deputy department heads could be holding the knife at the wrong angle or do something that he wasn't happy with, and he would call him an idiot, slap his hand as if he were a yeshiva boy, and he a reproachful rabbi.

Shaul, like all the other interns, had the job of being a "retractor," the person who holds the abdominal walls open so that the surgeon can work.

One day, when Shaul was holding the abdomen open but leaned in a little too closely to see what the professor was doing, his glasses fell off into the patient's gaping belly.

The room fell deadly silent. No one breathed, Shaul didn't dare to move, and everyone was expecting Prof. Marcus to react with humiliating shouts. Two nurses, as pale as their uniform, seemed to be on the verge of fainting. The assistant surgeon froze on the spot.

Shaul looked at Prof. Marcus and Prof. Marcus looked at Shaul, and after a short stare down, Prof. Marcus reached into the abdomen, took out the glasses, changed his gloves, turned to Shaul and said, "Change your gloves and come back."

Shaul changed his gloves and surgery continued as usual.

The professor didn't say another word about it, to the immense astonishment of everyone there.

Later, they all understood why he reacted so differently with Shaul. In Shaul's case it was a matter of force majeure, whereas with the nurses or doctors, their mistakes were due to negligence.

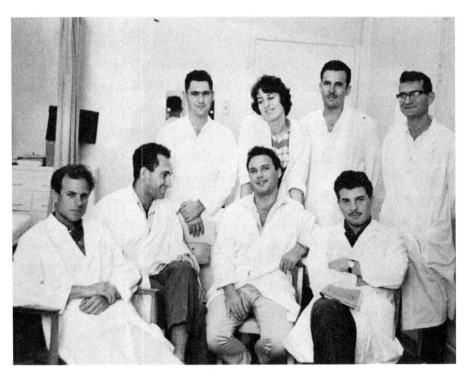

Shaul in the front row on the right with his fellow students

1966—TWO YOUNG DOCTORS ARE EXPOSED TO THE SECRETS OF REAL MEDICINE

At the end of 1965, the government was asking doctors to volunteer in border communities that were impacted by war. Shaul had just finished his internship. He and his good friend, Yehuda Shapira, decided to volunteer and were sent to the development town of Netivot. It cannot be denied that the relatively good pay also played a significant part in their decision. Shaul arrived with Dalia, who found work at the Dead Sea factories in Beersheba, while Yehuda came with his wife, Naomi, and their baby daughter.

The town's community was comprised of Moroccan Jews from the Atlas Mountains and Tunisians from Djerba, an island off the mainland. When they got there, they learned that the previous doctor had found ways to save time and provide care for all his patients: in order to finish his shift within a few hours, when he sometimes had to see a hundred patients, he would see 10 at a time. The 10 patients would go into his clinic, stand in a line with their mouths open so that he could check their throats, and then prescribe nose drops for one, give another sick leave from work, a third allergy tablets, and for the fourth—who he wasn't entirely sure what he was suffering from or how to treat him—he would immediately order an ambulance.

Throughout his time there, the doctor would call for at least two ambulances a day from Netivot to Beersheba, and usually for no justifiable reason. The doctors at Soroka Hospital would be furious.

Saying that, the fast-paced and amiable doctor was happy and kind-hearted. His patients would sometimes thank him with a sack of potatoes or a fine bunch of onions, and many would show their appreciation with homecooked food.

The two young doctors walked into this chaos without knowing anything about the previous doctor's practices. Although they were motivated, enthusiastic and idealistic, they were certainly inexperienced.

Shaul arrived at the clinic on his first day of work wearing his white robe and closed the door behind him, then waited for the first patient to knock. He was stunned when 15 patients stormed through the door, all of them making demands.

He stood up, asked them to leave the room, then went out to the waiting room and gave a restrained speech. He explained that from that day on, the procedures would be different, because order had to be maintained in the clinic. He told them that they had to come in one by one, not all at once. "I will receive only one patient at a time," he explained to the astonished crowd staring at him. "And you must knock on the door and enter only when I ask you to."

Shaul then turned around and returned to his room. Pleased with himself, he thought about how he'd been given the right to be both a doctor and an educator. No one knocked on his door, and all he could hear was silence.

Then, when he was considering getting up again to see why, the door burst open again and ten patients rushed in.

It's harder to educate people than it is to provide them with medical care, Shaul realized, and with some kind of parental instinct (although he did not yet have children), he got up, took off his robe, and left the room and then the clinic, muttering that he had no intention of treating any patients until they learned to respect his request.

They slowly understood, and not only accepted the new rules but also fell in love with him and Yehuda. For not only did the young doctors devote time to treating each patient, but they also showed a personal interest in them, not only in their medical issues. They knew what each of them did for a living, how many children they each had, they visited their homes and listened attentively to the community that was still acclimating to their new country.

One wintry night, Shaul was fast asleep after working continuously from morning to night, when there was a sudden loud and urgent knock on the door. "Come quickly!" they begged him. It was a couple who lived at the far end of town. They told him that someone at home was critically ill. Shaul noticed their grave expressions and terrible distress and realized that something awfully bad had happened. He tried to wipe the sleep from his eyes, quickly got dressed, picked up his doctor's bag and walked home with them in the dark, mud and cold. When he walked in, he was surprised to find the house crowded with worried people. It seemed like the entire neighborhood had come to support the suffering family. He looked around the room for the critically ill patient, but he didn't see anyone burning up with fever, or dying or screaming.

"Where is your patient?" Shaul asked.

Someone took his hand and led him to the other room. There, on a bright rug, lay a goat.

And indeed, she was in terrible agony and bleating loudly. A huge abscess on one of her udders was the source of her pain.

Shaul had no choice, and although he had no veterinary knowledge, he couldn't abandon the suffering goat or disappoint the dozens of pairs eyes staring expectantly at him.

He gave her antibiotics (albeit twice as much as needed) but the goat survived.

Shaul and Yehuda learned about customs with which they were unfamiliar. The young children, for example, slept in beds that their parents repurposed from orange crates. They washed the fruit and vegetables in the toilet and used the trash cans to store food. The farm animals lived together with them in their homes, but slowly but surely, the two of them began to look up to the people of the community, who were generous and warm and treated Shaul and Dalia, Yehuda and Naomi and their baby like family. They were invited to every bris, wedding and holiday celebration, had no choice but to watch the Indian movie that was screened every week in the community center (and were given front row seats). They learned about all the different kinds of couscous, and whenever Shaul and Yehuda stopped at the gas station to fill up, a crowd of people would always storm their car to wash it as a sign of gratitude.

And then there was their exciting motoring experiences.

Shaul and Yehuda were given and received a Susita Ducas, which was made of fiberglass. One time, when Shaul made a house call, he came out to find that local punks had broken off a piece of the car door. This made him terribly angry, and when it happened a second and a third time, he decided to hide behind a low fence and ambush them. To his amazement he saw no one, just a bunch of donkeys wandering about. It turned out that they were the perpetrators who enthusiastically and hungrily attacked the car and chewed off chunks of the fiberglass doors with their donkey teeth. They seemed to find it delicious. This happened time and again, and they slowly ate most of the door. When they could no longer close it, Shaul took string and rope and tied the pieces that the donkeys had been kind enough to leave them and drove off, imagining that his car was rattling over the Atlas Mountains...

The significant advantage of the time that Shaul and Yehuda spent in the remote development town of Netivot was the broad medical education that they received. They learned things they had not learned and would never have learned at medical school.

For example, they learned how to cure asthma by taking a cloth bag and filling it with prickly pears sliced into quarters and sprinkled with sugar. The sweet juice would drip into the mouth of the patient, who was thirsting for a cure, and sometimes—as the patients believed—it would cure them of severe asthma. They learned from the locals about the herbs they would boil and that

194

they solemnly swore contributed to the sexual potency of the men.

A few months passed and they received a call from Soroka Hospital asking why they weren't sending ambulances every day like before. Then a delegation from the central HMO office came, including the Southern District's head physician. They wanted to see the miracle for themselves and to try to understand how two inexperienced doctors had managed to create such perfect order in the infamously chaotic clinic, and to turn it into an efficient, professional and welcoming clinic.

To fulfill their need for culture, they would go to Beersheba, which was then a pioneer city with a fresh charm of its own. There they would meet impressive people who had moved down south to help in developing medicine and industry. They did this and although they were concerned about driving back to Netivot late at night, since it was near the Gaza Strip. It was 1966, before the Six Day War, and a relatively peaceful year in Israel.

1967–HADASSAH HOSPITAL ON BALFOUR STREET IN TEL AVIV (THE GIRL WHO ATE PLUMS)

At the end of 1966, Shaul received the good news he was hoping for: that he'd been accepted to specialize in pediatrics at Hadassah Hospital on Balfour Street in Tel Aviv, with the head of the department whose name went before him—Prof. Nahum Boger. Despite the charm of the city of Beersheba and the good reputation of the pediatric department at Soroka, he decided to return to Tel Aviv because he'd always set his sights on specializing there.

Shaul and Dalia moved in with her parents. They still had no children and Dalia continued to work for the Ministry of Industry and Trade. She traveled all week between Tel Aviv and Jerusalem.

It was a regular morning in Shaul's life as a pediatrics intern. The emergency room was bustling. Adults and toddlers lay side by side because in those days as the children and adults didn't have separate emergency rooms. Shaul was treating the children and babies, while right beside him, general practitioners were treating adults after a heart attack or performing emergency resuscitation.

Then a nurse came up to him and asked him to come quickly to help a patient. "She's not a child, she's 16-year-old, but she's writhing with terrible abdominal pain and there's no one to take care of her because the other doctors are dealing with emergencies."

He immediately went over to the girl to help her. Her parents looked terrified. Her father was biting his nails and her mother was prattling on and stroking her daughter's hand.

"Oh Doctor," the mother said, "my daughter ate a lot of plums and has a terrible stomach ache. I've never seen her like this before. Please examine her. We don't know what to do. She may have eaten too many, but should she be in so much pain?"

Shaul began to examine the patient carefully and thoroughly, who was moaning and shouting, when suddenly he noticed a cute little head appearing between her legs. The girl who had eaten the plums was giving birth.

The father's eyes almost popped out of his head in astonishment and indignation, and the doctor feared for the mother's well-being. At the last minute, the girl was transferred to the Kirya Hospital, where she gave birth to a sweet, healthy baby.

At that time, and at that hospital, the interns had to deal not only with the young patients, but also with their parents.

One morning, when he got to the emergency room, the nurse called him to check on a baby who had died of crib death. The baby was blue and not breathing at all. The young intern began doing CPR, trying to resuscitate the baby, and pressed over and over on his chest. When that didn't help, as a last resort, he injected adrenaline into the baby's heart.

There was no wall separating the rooms from the hallway, only a long glass window that people could look through and watch the doctors treating the patients.

When all of his attempts to resuscitate the baby failed, he was forced to declare the time of death and he went out into the hallway, where the father was waiting. Before he could utter a word, the father, who was a huge man and tremendously strong, started punching him.

Stunned, Shaul tried to defend himself, but the father was a mountain of a man and the tremendous rage he felt toward him made him even stronger.

"You killed my child!" he groaned, his voice heartbreaking. "I saw how you abused him and how you did it. I saw it all! How at first you pushed on his chest and then you injected something into his heart." The father lifted his arm to demonstrate, making it seems like the injection was used violently, like a sword. "Now I'm going to kill you," he continued before grabbing Shaul by the neck to strangle him.

Shaul tried to free himself from the father's strong grip, who had completely lost control, but the man was too strong, and he knocked him to the floor. The nurses started screaming for help but couldn't do a thing.

After a long, exhausting struggle, Shaul somehow managed to free himself from the father's grip. After catching his breath, he approached the angry father and mustering all his courage, said politely, "Come, let's go into the room for a moment and I'll explain exactly what happened and what I did."

And so, very patiently, Shaul explained what he'd done to try to resuscitate the baby, which were unfortunately all in vain.

Then the man began to cry and shriveled up in shame. He apologized and said that he'd lost his mind so badly that he could have killed him.

Shaul's heart ached for the father's loss and he reassured him that he understood; that it was indeed a real tragedy and he comforted him for his loss. It was a moment of extraordinary and moving human closeness for both men. And Shaul learned firsthand how healing a sensitive explanation could be for patients and their close ones.

As there were no sub-specialties yet in pediatrics, they received a broad education in general pediatrics and learned how to deal with critical situations, especially in the emergency room, where they worked day and night. Sometimes, they were on their own in the emergency room for hours on end, which sharpened their instincts greatly. Eventually, they could determine which of the 20 moaning children waiting in line was in urgent need of treatment. They could diagnose the children's conditions by the way they cried (the more they cried, the less critical their condition was). And they learned to differentiate between cries due to pneumonia, cries due to abdominal pain, or cries resulting from earache.

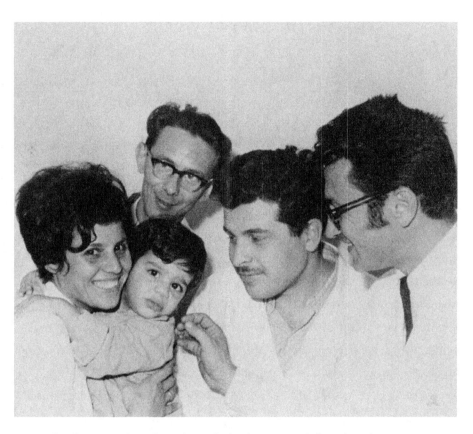

Shaul is second on the right with the late Dr. Rudich and Prof. Spirer at Hadassah Hospital in Tel Aviv

THE SIX DAY WAR

When Shaul began his residency in pediatrics in Tel Aviv, and he and Dalia moved in with Dalia's parents, they did so to save on costs, and it was also more convenient. Shaul got to enjoy his Jewish mother-in-law's cooking, and Yehudit happily fulfilled the role of mother, which he had lacked since he was a small child. The young couple, like their friends, were starting out on their professional paths. They were far from extravagant, and only went out to the few, good cafes that Tel Aviv had to offer. You could count the exclusive restaurants on less than one hand, including Casba and Gondola, where the important and influential people ate, such as Moshe Dayan, not paupers, which they were. There were still no movies on Friday nights in Tel Aviv, not to mention other shows, and there wasn't a single mall in all of Israel.

There was a recession and unemployment was on the rise. Morale was low and people were leaving Israel. The joke of the day was, "Whoever leaves the airport last is to turn out the lights."

Still, life in Israel was calm. That is, until the country was taken by complete surprise when the Straits of Tiran were closed, and the Egyptian army entered Sinai.

And then everyone waited, for a period that lasted about three weeks. People were nervous, worried if Israel would continue to exist, when only a mere 20 years had passed since it had been founded. It felt like there was another Holocaust on the horizon. The prime minister, Levy Eshkol, gave a stuttering speech to the nation, which only made everyone feel worse.

As he'd been so severely injured in the Sinai Campaign, Shaul had done only 18 months of duty, but in the meantime, he'd become a medical officer, and he now had the opportunity to finish his military service. To his great disappointment, for some reason, he wasn't called up, perhaps because of his disability. He would go to the Tel Hashomer base every day and implore them to recruit him. He, too, had been deeply affected (perhaps unjustly) by Eshkol's speech and he decided to initiate a meeting with Moshe Kol, whom he'd met when he was chairman of Youth Aliyah. He was now the Minister of Tourism for the Progressive Party. Shaul asked Kol to put pressure on the government to appoint Moshe Dayan as Minister of Defense; that the whole nation was hoping for it, as they had no faith in Levi Eshkol. Kol agreed with Shaul and was one of the ministers who in the end, recommended electing Dayan as Minister of Defense. Dayan would lead the war.

Just three days before the war broke out, Shaul was drafted and sent to Soroka Medical Center in Beersheba to wait for orders. He was to be posted wherever he was needed.

Shortly afterward, he received instructions to replace a doctor in the Arad area, who'd collapsed from the anxiety and stress. In the middle of the night, a driver took him to a *Hakash* (Elderly Corps) Battalion, made up of veterans of the War of Independence. It was the only battalion posted north of Beersheba, because as the IDF had no real intelligence regarding what to expect from the Jordanians, most of the army was deployed further south or up north.

The area was pitch dark and the driver couldn't find the battalion's location. They wandered for hours in the vicinity of Arad. Shaul was already sure he was going to be captured by the Jordanians, but fortunately, the guards noticed them before the Jordanians did. Although they almost shot them, at the last moment they noticed that they were driving an Israeli command car.

It was two in the morning, and at four-thirty, before Shaul had time to brief the paramedics, the Jordanians attacked them with a heavy barrage of fire. Some of their soldiers were wounded and required immediate medical attention. What Shaul didn't know was that the previous doctor hadn't given the medics any training in injecting morphine using real ampoules, and as such, they didn't know that the syringe had to be perforated in order for the liquid to come out. Only after the wounded men continued to scream in pain did Shaul realize that the morphine hadn't been injected and he corrected the problem. The area fell silent again shortly after the shelling, and it turned out that the Jordanian army had withdrawn (perhaps to defend Jerusalem).

Shortly afterward, the battalion received orders to advance toward Hebron. Theirs was the first battalion to "conquer" Hebron.

When they entered the city, they were surprised to see the streets empty and quiet. There wasn't a living soul on the street. Perhaps the Arabs of Hebron were afraid that the Jewish soldiers would attack them in retaliation for the riots of 1929. Suddenly, Shaul noticed a wounded little girl. He went over to her and saw that her head had been injured by shrapnel. They helped the girl into the command car and Shaul started cleaning her wounds and dressing them. One of the medics, who was a professional photographer, took a picture of the wonderful scene, and it became one of the most famous images of the Six Day War. It later appeared in the international press under the heading: "An Israeli doctor treats a Palestinian girl."

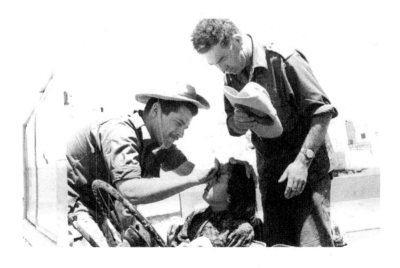

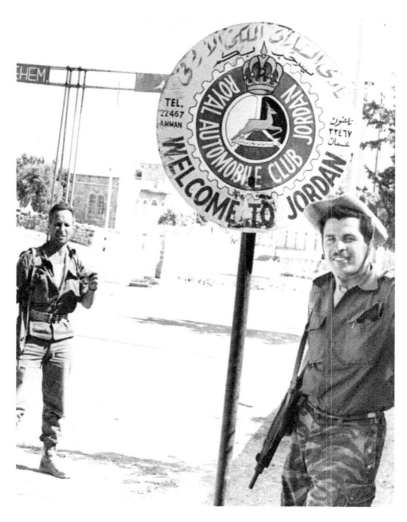

Shaul during the Six Day War

On the morning of the day that the Six Day War broke out, Dalia was on the bus on her way from Tel Aviv to the Industry and Trade office in Jerusalem, where she'd been working ever since they returned from Netivot. At the end of the previous week, Tel Aviv had filled up with soldiers, who were home on a break, and people felt that perhaps an agreement would be reached and that the war could be avoided. Dalia was reading Israel Beer's book, who foresaw the end of Israel in the "third round." (Beer was later arrested for spying). Looking out the bus window at the pine forests on the way to Jerusalem, Dalia wondered how long they would survive. It was only when she arrived at the office in Jerusalem that she heard that they were at war, and that Israel had already destroyed hundreds of Egyptian MiGs, their fighter jets. She was immediately sent home to Tel Aviv. But before she left, she called her former neighbor from 21 Washington Street, who asked her to come and visit.

"The Jordanians won't fight us," her friend stated with the certainty of an expert.

At 11:00 AM, when Dalia was about to leave her friend's place for Tel Aviv, all hell broke out and shells fell right by the building, near the border separating West from East Jerusalem. It was the Jordanians attacking them, and by so doing they decided the fate of the West Bank.

She had no choice but to spend three days and three nights in Jerusalem and bear the incessant noise from the bombings. Her parents actually took the news that she was close to the battle zone with relative calm, but everyone was worried about Shaul, who they hadn't heard from since he'd been called up.

On the first night, she sat on a small children's chair at the end of the shelter, which was crowded with the building's occupants. They had made makeshift beds for themselves, but she didn't get to shut her eyes. Dalia has always had a hard time dealing with sleep deprivation, and to her, not being able to sleep was a more serious threat than the bombs. And so, she found a solution: on the following nights, she went up to her friend's apartment on the first floor, took a mattress out into the hallway, pushed cotton balls deep into her ears, and slept soundly, as if her rest was being turned into a pleasant experience by heavenly music, not by booming cannons and mortars.

She was only able to leave her friend's place on Thursday afternoon, and was among the crowds who excitingly welcomed the soldiers as they moved through the streets in tanks and army vehicles. East Jerusalem had already been conquered, everyone was feeling euphoric, and the future looked bright. No one guessed that 50 years later, after the jubilee celebrations in 2017, after two intifadas in which thousands of Jews and Arabs were killed, and after the Oslo Accords, Israel would still be dealing with terrorist attacks, an occupation regime that is unacceptable to the world, the de facto division of Jerusalem, and the lack of any political solution on the horizon.

Dalia returned home to Tel Aviv hoping for some news from Shaul. There was nothing. It had been two weeks since he'd been drafted, and she had received no news. Dalia was extremely afraid and expecting bad news. Only on the eve of Shavuot (Pentecost), more than two weeks after he'd been drafted, Shaul called for the first time and reassured Dalia and her parents that he was well.

PROFESSOR BOGER—HEREINAFTER, "THE BOSS"

Shaul's initial fascination with play and with its healing abilities stemmed from his childhood experiences with his counselor Siegi Hirsch, who used imaginative play and laughter at the boarding school in Lasne after the war. But using play when conducting medical examinations was once again validated when Shaul was doing his residency in pediatrics at Hadassah Hospital in Tel Aviv. Prof. Nahum Boger, the son of the mythological principle of Herzliya Hebrew Gymnasium, Haim (Bograshov) Boger. Prof. Boger graduated from medical school in Montpellier, France, and belonged to the school that saw great importance in conducting a full physical examination of the patient, including of all clinical indications (tapping, listening to sounds, looking, observing, and more).

Prof. Boger was an artist when it came to examining young children. He knew how to keep them amused while he examined them, how to distract them and make them feel like it was all a game. Only rarely would they hear a child cry while Prof. Boger was examining them.

Everyone needs a good teacher, a mentor to guide them, and Shaul was lucky to have such a wonderful mentor. Prof Boger was happy to pass his magical wand onto Shaul, when he realized that his brilliant student was following in his footsteps. At first, however, it was difficult, because not only was he a brilliant doctor with vast knowledge in pediatrics, keen intuition and was quite knowledgeable, Prof. Boger was sometimes both mistrustful and critical.

The interns who worked under him and did the rounds with him would be amazed at both his expertise and the special bond that he so tenderly formed with the sick children, but they were afraid of his harsh criticism, which they would receive whenever he asked them a question that they couldn't answer. An intern who said something silly would turn as red as a beetroot when Boger looked at him dismissively and would then struggle to recover.

Prof. Boger didn't spend a lot of time in the department, but the time he spent doing rounds was so fascinating and significant that what Shaul and the other doctors learned from him was as vast and rich as the universe.

Prof. Boger had unique instincts, a sharp and discerning eye, and a brilliant mind that absorbed and processed all the information he was presented with in an instant. He could diagnose a child's medical problem with great precision. He would sweep through the department like a whirlwind, going from bed to bed, then stop suddenly by one of the children, look angrily at his interns and bark, "Didn't you notice that this child has pneumonia in the posterior lobe of his right lung?" He would conclude that just from the way the child was lying on one side, so that his other, healthy lung could breathe freely, as the other was clogged.

Prof. Boger may have been tough on the doctors he was in charge of, but he was as soft as butter with the children, and always played with them while he examined them. Shaul learned so many important things from him, such as how to avoid performing an invasive, usually painful lumbar puncture on children under two years of age who the doctors suspected may have meningitis. He learned to play with them (after bringing their temperatures down), even if they'd arrived with a burning fever and looked weak. Sometimes, by playing with the children, they would come to life, smile and start playing alertly, their apathy gone. That would rule out meningitis, along with its invasive and painful examination. And so, Shaul learned from Prof. Boger to incorporate play when performing an examination.

Shaul hoped to instill this method of examination in his own students, and thus avoid putting children through difficult and unnecessary tests.

"Medicine is much more than the total knowledge that the doctor accumulates," Shaul explained. "You can be a walking encyclopedia and still be a bad doctor. When you're dealing with a patient in the emergency room, you need to use all of your senses and instincts: sight, hearing, what the child looks like, if their eyes look focused, how they're looking at you, how they pick up toys, crawl, lie, breathe, sigh, and even cry. Over time, I've learned to distinguish between the different ways that babies cry, between a groaning baby in bad condition and a screaming but vital baby. And you, as the doctor, must watch the child, detect all the signs and symptoms and combine them in your mind while deciding what's important and what's not so that you can reach as accurate a diagnosis as possible. And you need to make logical sense of all the options you have, according to how prevalent they are, and only then can you know which tests to order and in which particular order, too, of course. This all has to be done very quickly. You learn all this in theory at medical school, but a large part can't be taught and depends on the personality and previous experience of each individual doctor. One of the most important tools that a doctor must have is empathy, for every patient but especially for children, who have very sensitive sensors and pick up everything, like dogs who can tell if you're afraid of them.

"Therefore, a doctor has to smile, show an interest in the patient and the patient's family, look them all in the eye, not at the computer, and explain patiently what is happening, without dashing their hopes."

Shaul's life circumstances contributed considerably to his empathy and abilities as a doctor with an extraordinary ability to reach the right diagnosis. The experience of being mortally injured during the war and his interactions with the doctor who gave him hope showed him just how powerful a doctor can be when treating a patient.

YES, YOU SURVIVED, BUT YOU WON'T BE ABLE TO HAVE CHILDREN

One heavy cloud hung over Shaul and Dalia's idyllic and happy marriage and Shaul's developing career.

Dalia was unable to conceive.

The gynecologist sent her for every possible test, and they all came out fine. It took two years for the doctors to send Shaul for tests. In those days, there was always a tendency to "blame" women first.

The doctor lowered his eyes and talked rapidly when he gave him the news, as if he wanted to get the job over with. Sitting in front of him was a fellow doctor, a Holocaust survivor who had been severely wounded in the Sinai Campaign, and had recovered, was married, studied medicine, and now had to give him the test results: Sperm Count—Zero. Shaul would not have children. That is, he could adopt, but he couldn't have children of his own.

Shaul turned as pale as a sheet as his inner world fell apart. He had been well trained in the hard life, but this blow was unbearable. Who doesn't want to start a family and have children, a continuing generation, a branch of himself to the future, and from there to eternity? But the young doctor, who had lost his parents, a brother and a sister in the Holocaust, had a special calling: to keep the family alive.

It also came as a severe blow to Dalia, when all of her friends had already given birth to their second child. Even the pregnant stray cats made her feel envious. It never occurred to her to abandon her husband, the love of her life, and she started weighing adoption.

Despite this, there was one word that Shaul hardly never used: despair. Without losing even a minute, the young couple began to go from one well-known gynecologist or urologist to another, but they all gave him the same answer and made crazy suggestions. One of them jokingly suggested, in poor taste, that they ask a neighbor to help. None of them offered any hope.

That is, until they met a doctor, who as if in a fairy tale, thought outside the box and tried to understand what could be causing the problem. It was Dr. Amnon Mor, an andrologist, and he diagnosed Shaul with a varicocele, or in other words, his veins were dilated. It turns out that following his injury in the war, an accumulation of blood vessels formed that were warming the area where the sperm flowed, and the warmth was damaging it before it could fertilize the egg. Dr. Mor believed that a spermatic vein ligation (an innovative operation at the time) could solve the problem. He gave Shaul the names of ten doctors from all over the world, and they all told him that he had nothing to lose, he could only gain.

And that's exactly what happened. Dr. Rakovchik, who'd operated on Shaul 12 years earlier, when he was wounded in the Sinai Campaign, now operated on him again, and two months later—as if by magic—Dalia was told that she was pregnant. Unfortunately, that pregnancy ended in a miscarriage, but they were delighted when two months later, Dalia fell pregnant again.

As they had started relatively late, Dalia and Shaul decided to have children without a break between, much like the ultra-religious who don't believe in contraception. Not many secular couples can boast that two of their children were born in the same year. Tali, their first daughter, was born at the beginning of 1969, and their second daughter Ronit, at the end of the same year.

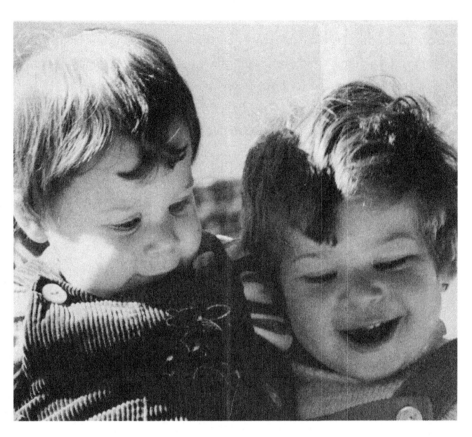

Tali and Ronit—almost twins

As the family was expanding, it had become time for them to put down roots somewhere, and Dalia and Shaul chose the Tel Ganim neighborhood in Ramat Gan. It was a quiet, green neighborhood of former, permanent military people that the villa hunters were slowly invading. Naturally, Shaul and Dalia could only afford to purchase an apartment, and they remained loyal to their first family home for 50 years. They both had to work hard for that apartment because they took out a huge mortgage. After her maternity leave, Dalia went straight back to fulltime work while Shaul, in addition to his shifts as a resident, and took on ten ambulance night shifts with Magen David Adom and got to know Israel's destitute.

Shaul had some rough experiences on those shifts, including delivering a baby in the ambulance and then tying the umbilical cord with shoe laces. It was an exhausting period for both Shaul and Dalia.

SPECIALIZING IN PEDIATRIC NEUROLOGY IN THE UNITED STATES AND THE YOM KIPPUR WAR

I WANT NEUROLOGY

Already in medical school, Shaul knew that he would specialize in pediatrics, a field that to him seemed more optimistic, due to the healing abilities and survival instincts that children are blessed with. He chose to take care of that stage in his life, even if it was repressed at the time, was still bleeding and cracked—his childhood.

In the last year of his residency in pediatrics, Shaul worked a great deal with Prof. Boger at the Child Development Center, which Prof. Boger initiated the opening of with help from the Joint as early as 1970. Shaul found himself drawn to neuroscience, with all its complexity, and began to think about the connection between brain activity and fetal development and then about newborns and child development. *It all starts in the head,* Shaul realized, *the brain controls all the organs of the body, both from a physical as well as a mental aspect, including our thoughts and emotions.* He decided that he wanted to specialize in brain neurology.

At that time, the field of pediatric specialties was still in its infancy, in the Western world in general and in Israel in particular. Adult neurologists didn't think there was a need for a separate field of pediatric neurology, because as far as they were concerned, they could treat children, too, even though the differences between children and adults is enormous. There had not yet been the explosion of information that there is today, and on their part, pediatricians believed that they could know all the fields they needed, from cardiology to neurology and more. They, too, thought that there was no need for subspecialties.

In the late 1960s, children were seen by general (adult) neurologists or by pediatricians interested in neurological problems. There were only a few pediatricians working specifically in neurology, but they hadn't received formal training. After an inspiring encounter in Jerusalem with Prof. John Menkes from Los Angeles, who was considered a genius and one of the top pediatric neurologists in the U.S., Shaul and his friend Yehuda Shapira decided that they wanted to specialize in pediatric neurology and child development.

As Shaul has always looked thoroughly into things, and after he took the opportunity to visit the U.S. for the first time, Shaul decided to take a month-long journey across the U.S. to find a suitable place to specialize, as there, too, the specialty began only in 1970.

After a fascinating journey all around the country, he decided on UCLA in Los Angeles, California, where Prof. Menkes happened to work.

Both Shaul and Yehuda were accepted to do their residency there. The two families were among the first of many Israelis to settle in L.A, and if they'd stayed, as some of their friends did, they would have certainly become elders of the community.

And so, Shaul set out on the long journey to fulfill his professional ambition and mental need. Was he aware of the fact that every time he saved a child, not only was he saving the soul of that child, but also an element of his own? Was that the source of his immense strength, which would make him do all that he could, never give up, go against the odds in order to save a child? Because that was what he did when he was dealing with cases defined as "lost causes"; with children who seemed to have only the slimmest of chances. Was that why he was so driven to achieve professional success, and become a leading expert in pediatric neurology in Israel? Was his success and deep and desperate desire for meaning and self-identity connected to his childhood? Was that the reason he so deeply identified with the children he treated, and is that where his sharp and unique intuition and creative and flexible diagnostic vision stem from? Shaul didn't choose to be just a doctor, he chose to be one who would shape the fate of children who had been dealt a bad hand right at the beginning of their life. It was at that point, just like his wonderful mentor, Siegi, that he would use his magical medical wand to bring back the smile on a child's face or put a smile on a child's face for the first time ever.

RESIDENCY IN L.A.– THE BEGINNING

Coming from Israel, which was a young developing country but already showing signs of neglect, to beautiful Los Angeles came as a shock to the Harels
and Shapiras. They were amazed by the well-kept streets, the grass strips along
the sidewalks, the exemplary cleanliness, the ornate and perfectly maintained
houses, the magnificent splendor of neighborhoods such as Beverly Hills and
Bel Air, the freeways, with four lanes on each side. They felt as if they'd arrived
in paradise, although admittedly, they did find it slightly boring. Before Dalia
started driving, she went for a walk with their two little girls, and she and
the postal worker were the only two people on the street. *What a waste*, she
thought to herself, *it's so beautiful and well-kept here, and for some reason,
everyone is in their cars.* The two families each had two daughters. They rented
apartments in the same building in Brentwood, a suburb in West L.A., and
helped and supported each other throughout their three years there.

When Shaul and Yehuda got to L.A., they found out that Prof. Menkes was
no longer the head of the department due to disagreements with the hospital's
management, but he was still conducting research and teaching.

Shaul and Yehuda, who'd expected a red carpet when they arrived at the
hospital to begin their fellowship year, or at least an organized reception and
a guided tour of the place, had a surprise in store: they were thrown right into
the cold water, in the best of tough American traditions. It was their first day,
but they were already expected to do consultations, and they had to find their

way to the pediatric wards on their own.

Despite their proficiency in general and emergency pediatrics, they knew almost nothing about neurology. On top of that, they also had a hard time understanding the medical records, as they weren't familiar with the typical American abbreviations. For example, FLK, which meant *Funny Looking Kids*, or FLP which meant *Funny Looking Parents*. There was no internet to look up what terms meant, only the Medicus Index, which they found themselves pouring over for hours.

The medical field in the U.S tended to be cruel. If a fellow were no good, the general pediatrics residents would ignore him. Only after six months of going home late after spending exhausting hours reading in the library could Shaul and Yehuda breathe more easily, because respect for them finally grew and they were called for consultations.

Still, they did have one advantage over the American fellows they were working with: the American school dictated that first they had to do all of the tests, and only then examine the child's clinical condition. The Israeli fellows had extensive experience in the emergency room and could identify a child's condition just from the way he or she cried and responded. They could tell the wheat from the chaff, and they worked according to the European school, which was more clinical and relied less on conducting supplementary tests. Also, the guidance they'd received from their teacher while doing their internship worked in their favor.

Shaul had developed a unique and playful way of examining a child in his earlier days of working in Israel, using a Raggedy Ann doll, which he found to be the most effective of all the dolls. Whenever he pulled it out, the children would be captivated by it, and sometimes it helped to avoid performing invasive tests on them.

This was in the early 1970s. The news on television was covering the demonstrations against the Vietnam War and Watergate. The music of Bob Dylan and John Baez was playing everywhere. The flower children were doing all they could to stay young, and even in their more strait-laced hospital social life, the two couples were sometimes offered a joint or bong.

FIRST CONSULTATION IN LA—ON THE FREEWAY

A number of amusing incidents happened to Shaul in the U.S.,, and his first encounter with the law was one of them.

The first thing the couples had to do was to buy a car. And Shaul found a great deal in the local newspaper—a red Pontiac with a sunroof and fancy white seats for just seven hundred dollars. As they say in Israel—America[6]. That evening, he rushed off to meet the seller, and after going for a quick spin, he handed over the money and bought the car. It did, however, have one downside: the air conditioner hadn't been installed, and was in the trunk of the car. The seller assured him that he could have it installed at any auto repair shop. Naturally, he believed the American, who made a wonderful impression. But Shaul went from one repair shop to another, and they all raised an eyebrow at him before refusing adamantly to take the job. In the end, he was sent by a car dealership to a repair shop out of town. He drove there with his friend Itche Weintraub, who had moved to L.A. a few months before them to do his fellowship in gynecology. Itche knew the roads, and he drove in front of Shaul to show him the way.

Soon after they set out, they heard a police siren, and Shaul was pulled over. Itche, unable to stop, continued driving. The police officer, as broad and tall as a barn door, got out of his car and walked toward him, his expression stern

---

6   In those days, America was seen by Israelis as the land of dreams.

and authoritarian. He looked somberly at the car papers and at the number plate and found four issues. He decided to take the car off the road, and Shaul couldn't do a thing about it. Then the officer noticed his international driver's license, which stated that Shaul was a doctor. As if by magic, the serious look on his face was replaced with respect and admiration.

"Are you a doctor?" he asked.

"Yes," Shaul responded. "My friend and I are fellows at UCLA."

The officer leaned over and asked in a soft, embarrassed voice, "Can I consult with you?" And then added, "A few days ago, I slept with a girl, and I have a discharge from my penis. Should I take antibiotics?"

A pediatric neurology fellow wasn't exactly the right person to ask, but then Itche appeared at the top of the hill and shouted, "Shaul, where are you?"

Shaul shouted back "Itche, come quickly, I've been asked for medical advice in a field that you know far more than I do!"

Itche came down and told the officer how to deal with his problem.

What a crazy thing: giving venereal disease advice to an American police officer on the freeway. And the officer was so grateful that he gave them a police escort to the repair shop, using his siren to clear the road for them. To Shaul's disappointment, this repair shop, too, couldn't think of a way to install the air conditioning, and he finally concluded that he'd been swindled.

He decided to try out the American justice system, and sued the seller in the small claims court, a wonderful invention in the eyes of Israelis in those days, which Israel didn't have until a few years later.

The American justice system proved itself. Shaul, who represented himself in his rather broken English, won the lawsuit and received double the amount he'd paid for the car as compensation. And thus, together with the true value of the defective car, which was only four hundred dollars, he could buy a reliable car with air conditioning that served them for their entire time in L.A.

TALI, WHEN A BROKEN HEART IS MENDED

Shaul realized there was a problem. The medical staff standing around Dalia's bed right after she gave birth to Tali, their oldest…after all the difficulties that they'd had…were whispering to each other. The head of the department was there to examine the baby, and his face looked serious.

Tali, a plump, sweet and beautiful baby, had been born with a heart murmur and they suspected a congenital malformation in her heart.

Because advanced imaging technology had not yet been invented in 1969, the doctors didn't know what exactly was wrong with her heart.

The only test that could be conducted in those days was cardiac catheterization, but since it was dangerous, the doctors preferred not to do it on such a young age newborn. After all their difficulties in starting a family, Shaul didn't want to worry Dalia and didn't tell her about the problem.

But on one hot summer day, when Tali was three-and-a half months old, she started crying uncontrollably and turned blue, leaving him no choice but to tell Dalia, who found the problem terrifying. She was already pregnant with their second daughter, Ronit.

Tali underwent catheterization when she was two-and-a-half years old, before they left for Shaul's fellowship in the U.S., and that's when they learned that she had a rather complex heart problem.

One of the reasons that they went to the U.S. was so that Tali could have open heart surgery at the Mayo Clinic in Rochester, Minnesota. Prof. McGoon was one of the best at the time, and he had a success rate of more than ninety-five percent. In Israel, the success rate was barely fifty percent.

On their way to L.A., they went to the Mayo Clinic for further tests, where they were told that because her heart was so small, they could only perform surgery when she was four years old. Today, it can be performed on one-week-old infants.

This made their time in L.A. incredibly stressful. Tali, who was an alert and happy little girl, would sometimes suffer from shortness of breath and turn blue. Dalia had to keep a constant eye on her while Shaul was at work.

Gili, who wasn't planned and came as a surprise, was born at the end of 1972, before Tali's vital surgery, and his name fitted him well. Gili, which means joy, lived up to his name and brought plenty of happiness to the family.

They held Gili's bris at the home of their good friends, Ziva and Ephraim Yavin, and they invited the whole small Israeli community.

In January 1973, in the middle of winter, they again went to snowy Rochester, Minnesota, and they took all the children with them. Dalia's mother, Yehudit, flew in from Israel, leaving Israel for the first time in 38 years. It was hard to imagine how such an inexperienced woman with broken English could be calm enough to handle three flights all on her own, the last in a small plane to the snowy area that reminded her of her homeland, Poland.

In January 1973, Tali successfully underwent the complex surgery. Dalia and Shaul will never forget how moved and relieved they were to see her lips and nails pink after surgery.

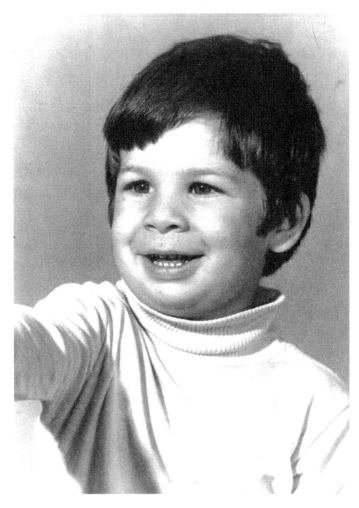

Gili at about a year old.

1971–LOS ANGELES, BECAUSE IT ALL STARTS IN THE HEAD

That morning, when Shaul was doing the rounds as a neurological consultant, examining the babies and children in the pediatric ward at UCLA, he noticed a lot of activity around one of the beds.

When he joined the crowd, he noticed a baby who was constantly having convulsions. As a neurology fellow, he'd been asked to examine him. He was told that the baby had been diagnosed with a heart defect, which was causing heart failure. The doctors standing around the baby felt helpless because they couldn't understand why the medication that they'd prescribed was having no effect on him at all.

The baby's condition was getting worse by the minute and his condition was becoming life-threatening. Because he was convulsing so badly, Shaul thought that the diagnosis may be incorrect. During his short time as a pediatric neurology fellow, he'd learned that when conducting a pediatric neurology examination, one should listen to the skull using a stethoscope. To the astonishment of all the doctors, he placed the stethoscope on the baby's skull, and nodded seriously to himself when, as he'd expected, he heard noises similar to a locomotive. He immediately realized that the baby had a vein of Galen malformation (VOGM) in the brain. In other words, the arteries in his brain were connected directly to the veins instead of to the capillaries, which help to slow the blood flow. The blood was rushing into his veins and then into his heart, thus causing it to be strained. Shaul could hear the blood whirling in the baby's brain.

That was why the baby's heart was failing. Shaul explained to the other doctors that they can detect vascular malformations in the brain by listening to the skull with a stethoscope, because sometimes the source of the problem is the brain, not in the heart. If they didn't correct the malformation in his brain, they wouldn't be able to treat the problem in his heart.

It was a simple examination, but no one had thought of doing it. Because of the new and accurate diagnosis, the baby was taken immediately to the operating room and his life was saved. As a result, Shaul became the talk of the day.

Years later, Shaul would teach all the doctors he trained to perform this simple and life-saving examination. He would require every doctor in the pediatric neurology clinics and child development centers that he managed to place a stethoscope on every child's head, at least once. Quite often, when Shaul examined children in this way, the children would turn to their parent and tell them that the doctor was confused, because he put the stethoscope in the wrong place.

Shaul came across more of such cases in his professional life, and when years later he would run into the parents of these children, they would remind him of his diagnoses. Years after he retired, a woman came up to him in a restaurant and greeted him warmly, then reminded him that she was the mother of "the boy with the beeping head." Shaul remembered the story. One day, the mother was hugging her six-year-old son, her head touching his, and she was surprised to hear a rather loud noise coming from his skull. Alarmed, she ran to their pediatrician, who referred her to Shaul.

She reminded him that when he heard the story, he became excited and said enthusiastically that detecting a murmur in the head with a hug is very rare.

He immediately held his stethoscope to the boy's skull and heard a rather loud noise, like a locomotive, which he immediately presented to the group of American students who were doing the rounds with him. Catheterization of the head made it clear that there was a malformation in the structure of the blood vessels, which was causing the blood to whirl around. After consulting with a number of experts in the U.S., Shaul decided not to operate on the child. The child grew up, the noise grew weaker, and possibly the twists that were slightly stopping the blood from flowing straightened out as he grew. But the mother, who at the time was very frightened, always remembered Shaul's soothing and relaxed tone, and valued the time he took to discuss the problem with experts abroad.

THE NEXT STEP IN THE FELLOWSHIP

The salary of a doctor doing his fellowship in those days was low, and the young families had to find a way to get through the month. Having no choice, they started moonlighting. Shaul was over the moon when he found a job doing shifts at a sports stadium. He got to attend all the exciting college basketball games, and that was when the university's team was first place in the country, with famous players such as Bill Walton. He got to see Bob Dylan, John Denver and Joan Baez live before a crowd of lively students, and sometimes he would bring along an Israeli friend or two. As commonly happens all over the world, the Israeli community in L.A. was very closely-knit, and most of them actually returned to Israel, where they remained friends.

They usually spent their leisure time having picnics in the parks, hiking in nature along the West Coast, and if they went away, they stayed at simple motels, some of them shady. Their friends became like family, and they celebrated the holidays together. On Purim, all the Israeli children would walk through the neighborhood in fancy dress, and their non-Jewish neighbors would look at them in bewilderment.

The news from Israel wasn't always good. Sometimes there were terrorist attacks, which would upset them deeply, such as the attack on Ben Gurion Airport, the attack in Ma'alot, and others. Still, the young families tried to focus on work and on enjoying the small things in life that the U.S. had to offer, being relatively peaceful and affluent compared to Israel.

At first, Shaul and Yehuda were planning to stay in L.A. for two years to complete their specialty in pediatric neurology. After the two years were almost over, Prof. Menkes convinced them to do another year, in adult neurology, so that they could be eligible to take the American Council for Higher Education board exams. For that, they needed to do two years in pediatric neurology and a year in adult neurology. Then they could return to Israel as American specialists and establish the field in Israel from scratch.

Since UCLA didn't have any spots in their adult neurology department, they moved to the University of Southern California (USC) hospital, which was an hour away from home. Since USC was a public hospital served a completely different population, which included drug addicts, alcoholics and rapists. Patients sometimes spat at them and working there could be quite traumatic. Prisoners were sometimes hospitalized there, and Shaul and Yehuda would have to examine them with a police officer present. But the medical staff, under the head of the department Prof. Joe Van Der Meulen, was excellent, and they welcomed the young doctors, who freed up some of their time to continue their research.

Receiving certification from the American Board of Pediatric Neurology was no easy feat, since under American law, only someone with a doctor's work permit from one of the states could receive accreditation for a medical subspecialty. Therefore, in order to take the specialty board exams in adult neurology, psychiatry and special skills in pediatric neurology, they had to first and foremost get an American work permit.

This meant that after three years of fellowship in the U.S., the two Israeli doctors had to take all the medical exams again, including those they'd passed years before in Israel. They had to study all the material again and be tested on it!

OCTOBER 1973–THE YOM KIPPUR WAR

It was a routine Saturday in the Harel family's home in L.A. Yom Kippur (the Day of Atonement) had already begun in Israel, but unlike in Israel, in L.A. the traffic didn't stop moving, and bicycles and children didn't stop racing about on the streets. The air didn't carry that sacred silence.

Then the phone rang. It was eight in the morning. Their friend Shuka, who had done his fellowship in pediatric nephrology in New York, was on the line.

"Dalia, guess what happened?" he said, his voice animated.

"What happened, Shuka?" Dalia asked, her voice still drowsy with sleep.

"Syria and Egypt have invaded Israel."

Dalia almost fainted and jumped out of bed.

Shaul wanted to leave immediately for Israel.

"Forget it," Shuka said confidently. "There's no reason to go. It'll all be over within a few days. We just have to surround them and then give them a fatal blow."

Three days later, Shaul was on his way to Israel.

In those three days, Shaul did another never-ending shift at USC.

During one of his few breaks, when he passed by a television, he stopped, glued to the spot, refusing to believe the images of captured IDF soldiers sitting in the sand, their hands behind their heads. As if what he was thinking wasn't bad enough, he suddenly recognized one of the soldiers, who must have been serving as the battalion doctor.

By the time night fell, Shaul knew deep in his heart that he had to return to Israel. He felt that the country was in a critical situation, and he knew clearly that he couldn't continue his fellowship, shifts and his life in America.

The next day, Shaul asked to meet with the Prof. Van Der Meulen, whom Shaul so admired and liked.

"I'm sure you've heard about what's going on in Israel," Shaul said. "I can't continue my fellowship right now, with my home in flames."

Prof. Van Der Meulen stared inquisitively at Shaul. "Have you been called back?" he asked.

"No," Shaul said, "but that's how I feel."

"Are you leaving your family here?" asked Prof. Van Der Meulen.

"Yes, for now," responded Shaul

"I see," said Prof. Van Der Meulen, and after a short pause he added, his tone serious. "Do me a personal favor, Dr. Harel: when the Egyptians shoot, lower your head."

Shaul smiled.

"And I want you to know that even if it takes a month or two, or even six, I'll keep your fellowship spot for you, and I'll also keep paying your salary to your wife," Prof. Van Der Meulen told Shaul in a confident yet comforting tone.

Stunned and moved, Shaul went home to Dalia, knowing that if she didn't give him her blessing, he wouldn't be able to go.

Dalia looked at their three young children: Tali, who was four-and-a-half; Ronit, who was three-and-a-half; and Gili, who was just 13 months old. She sighed and said to Shaul, "You can go, I'll be fine."

Yehuda received Naomi's blessing, while she, too, remained in L.A. with their three kids. Her youngest son Itai was Gili's age. Was it because they were only 32 years old, young enough not to comprehend the danger? Or the belief that Shaul and Yehuda would be serving at the hospital?

The embassy contacted a couple of Jewish doctors, who willingly donated their plane tickets to Shaul and Yehuda.

In the meanwhile, the airlines had stopped flying from the U.S. to Israel, and the only way to get there was on an El Al flight from London carrying weapons and medical staff to Israel. Shaul and Yehuda flew to London, and went to the Pan Am hangar, where thousands of Israelis from all over the world were trying to catch flights back to Israel. The airport staff asked if someone was handing out gold there.

Shaul tried to get on a flight but orthopedic, plastic, and other surgeons had priority, not pediatricians. In the end, his stubbornness paid off, and he was allowed to board. Most of the passengers sat on the floor singing Israeli songs, as if they were off to a big party.

On the plane, he met other kinds of volunteers, such as the Israeli man to his right, who was a paratrooper medic and had left the country for Denmark twelve years previously, where he'd opened a small restaurant. When he heard that war had broken out, he dropped everything to go back to Israel. On his left, there were two plastic surgeons from Chicago.

But nothing prepared him for what would happen at Ben Gurion Airport: there in the blackout, was a long line of hundreds of cars waiting for them outside the airport. They were older volunteers who were offering to take the volunteers from abroad anywhere in the country. Shaul's eyes filled with tears at that Israeli camaraderie, and he felt at home again.

Every day, he went to Tel Hashomer Hospital hoping to be posted somewhere, but things were crazy and disorganized. Meanwhile, they asked him to help in the emergency room, where they were admitting the wounded. The things he saw were hard to bear…severely burned soldiers who had been trapped in burning tanks, and a steady and endless flow of badly wounded soldiers. There was a pervasive feeling of despondency.

Finally, he was ordered to go south to Refidim Base, which was about 12 miles from the Suez Canal and where the IDF had their biggest logistics camp. He was to replace the doctor there, who was exhausted from the pressure.

It wasn't the crazy new routine, which included training with the regular paramedic team, nor treating the wounded or jumping into trenches when the Egyptians bombed the camp (sometimes twice a day) that made Shaul down; it was the lack of equipment (he was given a Czech rifle) and food, the negligence, and even the corruption that he was witness to now and again.

The base commander, who didn't like Shaul's critical view of the situation in the base (for instance, the team had no experience in using morphine injections), tried to get rid of him.

He was handed the opportunity when one day, an army radio crew arrived at the base that had been sent to cover the front lines.

"Dr. Harel," the commander said, "why don't you accompany the crew? Take your bag and get into the jeep."

Shaul found himself in the jeep with a photographer and two reporters, passing the Suez Canal as it was being heavily shelled and looking in amazement at the dozens of tanks that were stuck in the sand and at the utter chaos in the field. Suddenly, Egyptian MiGs attacked the convoys (and Shaul and the reporters who were stuck with them). It was a hair-raising experience, even for Shaul, who had taken part in battles during the Sinai Campaign, when he was severely injured.

Eventually, the jeep managed to infiltrate and cross the canal, and he went with the reporters to all the army outposts on the front lines, where they interviewed Arik Sharon and took the famous photo of him with the bandage around his head.

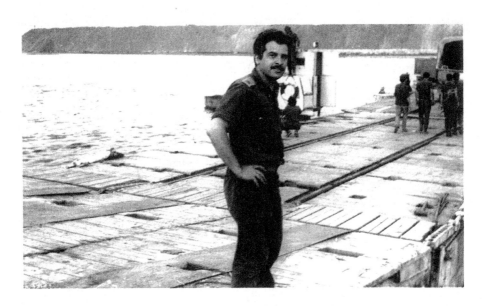

Shaul on the bridge over the Suez Canal

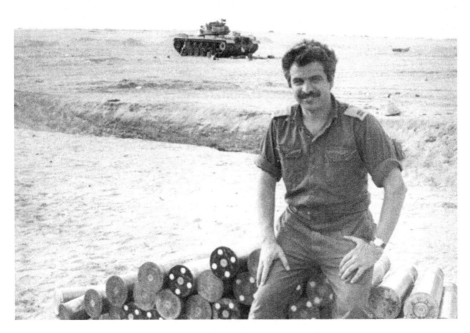

Shaul after crossing the Suez Canal

Dalia and Naomi were left on their own in L.A. with the kids for more than a month, keeping each other's spirits up in light of the bad news reports on the war against the Egyptians, which were shown on American TV, but were censored in Israel. They felt terribly alone and found it exceedingly difficult to continue life as usual. On top of the stress, Dalia felt insecure, living on her own with three young children in an apartment in L.A., a city that at the time was not crime free. She came up with a simple solution: every night, she placed the broomstick between the door and the door handle, which helped her to feel safe. Plus, to fall asleep, she would drink half a glass of Southern Comfort, which she later found out was whisky that had been upgraded with sugar.

On occasion, she would call Israel and be surprised by her parents' and the public's complacency. As the home front wasn't being attacked, and there were no reports or broadcasts from the field, no one really knew the growing number of casualties and wounded, or how serious the situation really was. In the U.S., on the other hand, they were constantly broadcasting footage from the war, and the situation seemed dire. Dalia was very anxious and worried, mainly because Shaul had no way of calling her parents and they hadn't talked, which meant that they couldn't tell her how he was.

But one day, Dalia finally received a sign of life from her husband—when Shaul popped up on Israeli television! He was sitting on a tank on the other side of the Canal, calmy eating an apple. Excited and relieved, Dalia's mother immediately let her know.

Shaul was away from home for a month-and-a-half, after which he returned to L.A. with Yehuda to continue their fellowship. When the two walked into the department at USC, they were received with welcome back and peace signs.

A few weeks later, Shaul was asked by the United Jewish Appeal (UJA) to give a talk to Jewish American doctors about the medical side of his experiences during the Yom Kippur War, with the aim of raising donations. Despite how hard he was working and his moonlighting jobs, Shaul volunteered to give talks, and every weekend, he ran from city to city throughout California and Arizona, capturing the hearts of his audiences after painting a slightly pretty picture of the way Israel functioned during the war. After each lecture, the donations increased, much to the UJA's joy. After a while, the UJA suggested that Shaul turn his talks into a lucrative side business and offered him a commission of ten percent of the donations he raised. To their surprise, Shaul refused to accept compensation for his talks, and said, "I'll do this for as long as I can, because I have a commitment to my work and my family, but by no means will I take a commission, because it'll make me feel uncomfortable and I'll lose my honesty."

Shaul continued giving talks without taking a penny for himself. A few months later, he was astonished to discover that unlike him, others representing Israel in a formal capacity took what they were offered for the talks, and for giving their blessings at Bar Mitzvah celebrations.

After three-and-a-half fellowship years and hard work in the U.S., Shaul returned to Israel with almost nothing to his name. He had looked out for himself and his family, but more importantly—he was at peace inside.

RESEARCHING FETAL DISTRESS AND BRAIN DEVELOPMENT

In addition to doing his fellowship and the extra jobs that he had taken on, Shaul also continued to work on the fascinating study he'd begun on intra-uterine growth restriction (IUGR) at UCLA. The study had a live model—a rabbit that was used to simulate human situations. Prof. Van Der Meulen heard about Shaul's study and called him in to talk.

"Would you like to continue your research?" Prof. Van Der Meulen asked.

"Very much so!" Shaul replied. "But how can I, when I'm doing my fellowship in adult neurology, and I have to do a good job in the department?"

"Would you like to?" Prof. Van Der Meulen asked again, insistently.

"I sure do," Shaul replied, surprised.

"Then that's that," Prof. Van Der Meulen determined. "I'll take care of your work schedule."

Prof. Van Der Meulen spoke with the head of the gynecology department, Prof. Quilligan, and told him about Shaul's important study. Van Der Meulen explained that he was funding it, but as it was also related to Quilligan's field, he was hoping that he could give Shaul a place to work in his lab. Prof. Quilligan agreed.

Prof. Van Der Meulen gave Shaul a lab technician, and he continued his study. At the same time, he instructed the chief resident to replace Shaul while he performed surgery on rabbits.

That really upset the chief resident's, and he snapped angrily at Shaul, "You and your bloody rabbits!"

Vascular placental insufficiency can cause damage to a fetus' organs. When this happens, the fetus preserves the most vital organs for its survival, the heart and brain, and to do so, it uses a mechanism that dilates blood vessels to these organs and constricts blood vessels to less vital organs (such as the liver, kidneys and skin). This process is called *brain sparing*. If the placental insufficiency is severe and prolonged, the blood flow to the brain eventually fails and the brain is damaged. The condition can be detected with a color Doppler ultrasound, which estimates the blood flow in the brain and in the placenta's blood vessels. With the use of an equation, the blood flow index, the moment that the brain begins to suffer can be determined and the baby can be delivered early.

The gestational period is significant and critical for the fetus, because if the fetus is born prematurely, it can suffer damage, but on the other hand, if it stays too long in the womb, it can suffer from fetal distress and the brain's development can be retarded.

Shaul's goal was to find the optimal time to deliver a baby when intrauterine growth restriction (IUGR) is indicated.

How did he do this? He created a model using a rabbit to simulate human conditions in a state of IUGR to see how the rabbit kittens continue to develop after birth.

Shaul performed a caesarean section on the rabbit in the last trimester of her pregnancy (the gestation period of a rabbit is about thirty days), at a time when vascular placental insufficiency increases, similar to a pregnant woman with IUGR. A pregnant rabbit has a bicornuate duplex uterus, with embryos in each horn. There are fan-like blood vessels going from the uterine arteries to each fetal placenta. In one horn, Shaul and the technician tied 20 to 30 percent of the blood vessels, thus narrowing it and causing restriction and infarction, which reduced the flow of blood in the placenta of each fetus. In this way, they caused placental insufficiency, similar to what happens sometimes during a woman's pregnancy.

They left the second horn as it was, and the fetuses in that horn served as a control group. After the c-section, they closed up the rabbit's belly and allowed the pregnancy to continue. Five days later, on the estimated date of birth, they performed another c-section, removed all the baby rabbits from both horns and compared the two groups.

The indices that were studied included: body weight, head circumference and biochemical indices of the brain, such as the number of cells, myelin (the white fatty substance that envelops the cell fibers), axons, which are important for electrical conduction, as well as a number of receptors.

Shaul then repeated the experiment, except this time, when he performed surgery to narrow the blood vessels, he used subcutaneous color to mark the fetuses in the control group and allowed the rabbit to give birth naturally.

He observed the fetuses after they were born, conducted cognitive tests and neurological tests and found that at a month old, the rabbits from the restricted horn were hyperactive, had more symptoms of ADHD and were slower learners than the rabbits in the control group. As part of this study, Shaul developed an innovative index that was introduced into the scientific literature: the cephalization index, which is the ratio of head circumference to body weight. It is based on the principle of brain sparing and is used to express the severity of IUGR—the more severe the IUGR process is, the higher the index (brain circumference divided by body weight).

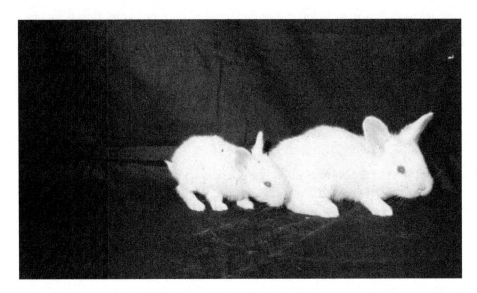

An IUGR research rabbit at 21 days, compared to the control

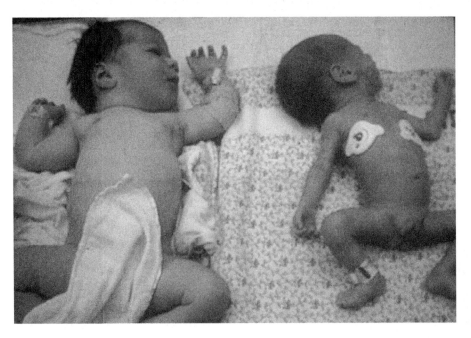

An IUGR baby (compared to a normal baby of the same age)

The conclusions of the study showed that there are clear significant differences between the fetuses that suffered from placental insufficiency and the "normal" embryos.

In other words, Shaul built a model that enabled the early diagnosis and detection of fetal distress. This was applied to humans by stressing the importance of preventing factors that lead to IUGR, such as preeclampsia, smoking, alcohol, drugs and bad nutrition, as well as the importance of early detection of developmental risks, which would allow them to treat fetuses and neonates earlier.

The fellowship was over, and the family was soon to return to Israel. Although it was clear to them that they were exchanging a promising financial future and relative security compared to a life in Israel of constant confrontation, they and a number of their friends didn't want to stay in the United States. And Shaul's personal history as a Holocaust survivor naturally played a significant part in his strong desire to return to Israel.

Before Shaul said goodbye to his job at USC, Prof. Van Der Meulen called him in again for a chat.

"As I see it," he said, "identifying and treating children at risk is an important field. As we have no experience in the field, and I know from the IUGR model that you developed using the rabbit that you have an interest in this field. I'd like you to continue working on this for a few more months so that you can apply the knowledge you acquired for USC."

He offered Shaul a scholarship for six months so that he could check out programs at the best centers in Canada and the U.S. and write a project according to which the clinical program would work to identify developmental disorders in fetuses and children at an early stage.

It was an opportunity of a lifetime; an offer that couldn't be turned down.

Shaul thought about how he'd be able to apply all that he learned; he did so later in Israel.

Dalia found herself once again in a difficult situation, but she agreed to a five-month separation from Shaul.

At the end of October 1974, Shaul accompanied her to New York, and she returned with their three young kids (including a two-year-old) to her parents in Israel, while Shaul stayed behind.

When she got off the plane with her children and saw her parents, she was so moved that she almost wanted to kiss the ground (after being away for three-and-a-half years). She felt almost like one of the Libyan immigrants that with whom Shaul had arrived in Israel.

It was a year after the Yom Kippur War, and the country she returned to was still in mourning. She saw relatives and people she knew who had lost their sons. Israel felt dull and poor compared to the glistening material paradise she had left in L.A. The most difficult question that she was asked now and then, and that sometimes made her toss and turn in bed, was "What did you come back for?"

Still, the move, which was difficult for her family, proved to be the right one.

Shaul spent the next few months preparing the project called "A practical model for early detection, assessment and treatment of neurodevelopmental disabilities," which included a program for integrating community services with medical center services. Until then, the main focus had been on school-age or near-school-age children, and the approaches to medical and para-medical intervention were disappointing, because there was no awareness that the children had by then reached the point of no return. All that they learned about the human brain during the 1970s shifted the focus of inter-est to intrauterine brain development and to the first three years of a child's life, the period known as the critical period in brain development. During this time, the brain is particularly sensitive to damage, but it is also flexible enough to enable intervention and therapeutic changes. In this time period, any detection of a disorder and its treatment has a decisive impact on a child's continued development and it can change the developmental prognosis.

In the 1970s, Shaul was aware that there was a lack of satisfactory community services for diagnosing children at risk, especially in low-income families. And this resulted in a vicious cycle that consisted of a few factors:

1. A close relationship between medical issues during pregnancy and early childhood and developmental problems;
2. A lack of developmental education for children growing up in deprived conditions, which contributed to the disabilities that they were born with and prevented compensation for moderate deviations in development, which can sometimes be overcome in an environment that IS optimal for the child;
3. A combination between poor organic factors and educational-environmental factors, which accumulate and lower the odds of the child bridging the gap and reducing it, reversing limitations, and thus they become irreparable.

As such, the purpose of Shaul's program was to propose a simple, practical model for early detection and intervention in infants and children with developmental problems, a model that would efficiently and cost-effectively combine medical services with community services. He envisioned it being applied at the parent and child centers all over Israel.

There is no doubt that formulating this program created the foundation for Shaul's expertise in diagnosing developmental disorders, discovering appropriate interventions, and more.

Five years after he returned to Israel, Shaul received another offer from Prof. Van Der Meulen, who called him in Israel and said, "I've been filling the position of vice president of health affairs for USC and chair of the committee selecting the head of pediatric neurology at the children's hospital in L.A. I'm offering you the position."

Shaul was extremely excited by the flattering offer, which undoubtedly meant a prestigious career with a very high salary. He knew full well that not only was the hospital considered one of the top ten in the U.S., and that it would place him at the forefront of global research, but that with Prof. Van Der Meulen at the helm, he would have an unlimited research budget at his disposal.

It was an offer that seemingly, he couldn't refuse. But both Dalia and Shaul knew that accepting the offer meant immigrating to the U.S. They weighed the pros and cons, but their desire to live in Israel tipped the scales. From the very beginning of his professional career, Shaul had decided that his goal was to promote pediatric neurology in Israel and to put it on the global map, and so, even this tempting offer didn't sway him from what he saw as his purpose in life.

Two weeks later, Shaul called Prof. Van Der Meulen and told him, "I'm very touched by your proposal, but as a Holocaust survivor, I feel that my place is in Israel, and I want to advance pediatric neurology and child development there. There is plenty of work to do."

Prof. Van Der Meulen understood and wished him the best of luck.

Many years later, in 2013, things came full circle, when Dalia and Shaul screened *Children Without a Shadow* in L.A. (the film that Belgian television and the Darden brother produced). Shaul had also been invited by the USC Department of Pediatric Neurology to be a visiting professor and to lecture on the vast and important research he conducted on fetal distress, which he continued at the Weizmann Institute after he returned to Israel. Shaul asked that Prof. Van Der Meulen be invited, and although he had Parkinson's, his mind was still just as sharp, and he came with his entire family. They hadn't seen each other in 40 years, and their eyes became damp when they saw each other. Shaul opened the lecture with a story about the study on rabbits that Prof. Van Der Meulen insisted he do and noted that it was thanks only to him that he had the opportunity to advance and develop the field. He spoke about how Prof. Van Der Meulen allowed him to return to Israel during the Yom

Kippur War and supported him and his family. He added everything that Prof. Van Der Meulen did for him afterward, too.

The silence in the hall was touching, and then suddenly there was a wild round of applause.

Shaul broke out in a smile, thankful that he had been given the opportunity to thank Prof. Joe Van Der Meulen while he was alive.

THE BATTLE TO ESTABLISH PEDIATRIC NEUROLOGY AND CHILD DEVELOPMENT AT THE TEL AVIV MEDICAL CENTER AND IN ISRAEL

RETURNING HOME AND ESTABLISHING MODERN PEDIATRIC NEUROLOGY IN ISRAEL

The family moved back into their modest apartment in Tel Ganim in Ramat Gan and set off on their new path in life. Dalia started working as an economist for the Ministry of Agriculture, trying—as the true city person that she was—to fit into a world that was completely foreign to her. She loved her work, the fascinating tours, as well as the interactions with agriculturists working the land. Most of them were idealists, and they shared touching stories. She participated enthusiastically in implementing the agricultural reforms that began at the end the 1980s and which were committed to a more realistic outlook, such as reducing the subsidies of hundreds of millions of dollars that were a burden on the state budget. The tough production arrangements were made more flexible, and the manufacturing industries were streamlined. She loved the discussions and the long debates with the agriculturists and with the people from the budget department. She was soon seen as an objective party who could mediate between the farmers and the Ministry of Finance. She continued working for the ministry until she retired after 25 years, 11 of which she held the senior positions of vice president and deputy CEO.

But in addition to her work at the Ministry of Agriculture and her full-time position of mother of three, she also gave Shaul her full support so that he could devote all of his time to work and research and reach the heights to which he aspired. In a way, she was just spoiling him. She did all the shopping, cooking, paid the bills, renovated the apartment, and took care of everything. She had hardly any paid help because government salaries have never been high. Grandma Yehudit, who was extremely devoted to her family, was of great help. Shaul certainly felt a great deal of affection for her, loved the delicious food she cooked for them and made sure to ask how she was every day. After Dalia's father died, Yehudit spent every weekend with the family and joined them on their trips in Israel and abroad.

In the late 1960s and early 1970s, the standard of medical care in Israel from a specialization point of view was not yet as good as in the U.S. While in the U.S. there were already subspecialties in pediatrics, they didn't yet exist in Israel. There was no genetics, nephrology or cardiology then…not even pediatric neurology.

And so, when he returned from his fellowship in L.A., Shaul went back to work in the Ichilov Hospital's pediatric department as a senior pediatrician, hoping to apply the knowledge he'd acquired in the U.S. But it wasn't all that simple.

The older neurologists, particularly the department head, treated him with suspicion and claimed "there is no such thing as pediatric neurology. There are neurologists and there are pediatricians with an interest in neurological problems." At the same time, the pediatric department didn't know him yet, and the pediatricians continued to consult with the adult neurologists. Shaul tried to insist, but the head of the neurology department was more insistent and said, "If you want to see pediatric cases in neurology, please be so good as to join the adult clinic, where you can see children. I can't give you exclusivity on consultations regarding hospitalized children in the pediatric ward, even when there may be a neurological problem. You can join the adult neurology consultation team and see children in that framework."

Shaul weighed his options: he could argue with the "omnipotent" head of the neurology department and risk having him go against him with full guns blazing and of being prevented from developing a neurology service for children, or he could take his advice and prove through his work that he is better (certainly than the adult neurologists), succeed because he excelled, and wait slowly and patiently for things to change.

"Okay," Shaul said to the department head. "So you'll let me work at your clinic? I accept your offer gladly."

And that's how it was. Shaul started examining children, and since he came from the American school, where it was customary to conduct comprehensive and thorough tests, talk to the parents as required, right down an orderly consultation, with a differential diagnosis, and so on, he acted accordingly. The result was not long in coming: slowly but surely, all the parents demanded to see only Dr. Harel for a neurological consultation for their children. And slowly but surely, the pediatricians from the pediatric ward also wanted only Dr. Harel's medical opinion, because he would take the time to sit with them and explain to them exactly how he'd reached his diagnoses.

Shaul did another thing: he willingly helped and gave advice to anyone who wanted it. He traveled all over the country giving talks on pediatric neurology, and even became a guest lecturer at Tel Aviv University. He slowly gained a reputation as an expert in pediatric neurology, especially in the central Tel Aviv region. After a great deal of pressure was put on him, the head of the neurology department called Shaul at the end of the year and told him that it was time to talk. "Look," he said, "you see all the kids with neurological problems, so okay, as far as I'm concerned, you can open your own clinic."

Shaul was lucky, as the head of the Tel Aviv Medical Center at the time was Prof. Arie Harel (no relation), and he was the former Israeli ambassador to Russia and Romania. He was an endocrinologist, a leader in his field in Israel, and a man of vast knowledge. He liked Shaul very much, and when the opportunity arose, he put Shaul in charge of pediatric neurology services in the pediatric department, which was still located at Hadassah Hospital in Tel Aviv, even though it was part of the Tel Aviv Medical Center.

It was 1976.

Quietly and pleasantly, without any arguments, Shaul started one of the first pediatric neurology services in Israel. Yehuda Shapira began to establish the pediatric neurology unit at Hadassah Mt. Scopus Hospital in Jerusalem. At that time, a group of leading pediatric neurologists was emerging in Israel. They had all specialized in the U.S., including Yehuda Shapira, the late Rafi Weitz, Nathan Brand, and Nathan Gadot, and in 1976, they founded the Israel Pediatric Neurology Society.

Other than running the pediatric neurology service, Shaul also started working at the Child Development Center, and when Prof. Boger retired, Shaul was put in charge of the institute, which belonged to the Tel Aviv municipality's public health department.

CREATING A REVOLUTION, THE SMART WAY

One of Shaul's jobs was to promote awareness in community health services of developmental neurological issues and to introduce growth charts for babies and children at Tipat Halav centers (family care centers for parents, babies and children).

It wasn't that easy.

In the 1960s, Tipat Halav and other family health centers fulfilled only two roles: vaccinating babies, and teaching mothers about breastfeeding and nutrition. No developmental follow-up was done, including growth curves. Shaul contacted the head nurse of Tipat Halav and suggested using growth, measurements and developmental tests for all babies and children to monitor their development and ensure that they were on the right track.

He received a chilly and anxious response, and the head nurse claimed that the nurses were very busy, that they weren't public health clerks, and that they didn't have time to fill in weight, length and head circumference data in growth curves. Marking the points on the growth curves is a secretarial job, and the psychological and developmental tests are the psychologists' business.

Shaul didn't argue with her. He realized that her anxiety could be circumvented in only one way. He wanted the nurses themselves to have an insight into the immense importance of monitoring growth and development, and so he developed a course that he gave to the Tipat Halav nurses in Tel Aviv.

In the course, which was on the basics of child development, Shaul revealed the fascinating mysteries of the brain, introduced the connection between tracking normal growth and the ability to prevent abnormalities and developmental disorders, and to treat them in a timely manner. He also showed them how easy it was to monitor the babies and children.

The nurses were quick to respond. They went to the head nurse and put a great deal of pressure on her, claiming that they now understood the importance of detecting deviations in development. They realized how important, diverse and challenging their work could be.

Then an argument broke out over where the first pilot would be, and the rest is history. Today, the development and growth of every baby in various fields, is strictly measured, recorded and marked on a growth chart. These are vital to developmental monitoring, and developmental screening tests such as the Denver test are used.

It should be said that in the 1970s and 80s, Tipat Halav was still an institution that Israel could be proud of and that could serve as an example throughout the world. Their contribution to detecting problems in early childhood was significant, particularly in the lower socio-economic groups.

Years later, Shaul was devastated when he foresaw their decline, which resulted from a lack of budget, their lack of suitability to the growing number of children, and they were shuffled between the Ministry of Health and the medical health funds.

1981—A YEAR IN NASHVILLE TENNESSEE, MAJORING IN COUNTRY MUSIC AND AMERICAN BOARD EXAMS

In the summer of 1980, the Harel family took a break, and again, in the best of tradition, took another year with the Shapira family in Nashville, Tennessee, the capital of country music, which Shaul loved.

Shaul and Yehuda needed to take the American Board of Pediatric Neurology exams and were accepted to the Vanderbilt University Medical Center in Nashville. It was a private hospital that had public hospital downtown with which it was affiliated, where they treated children from lower income families. Their plan was to take the exams and return to Israel to establish pediatric neurology in Israel as a specific specialty.

Once in Nashville, they both began working in the pediatric neurology clinics at Vanderbilt Hospital and at the hospital downtown, and at the clinics for adults (because the board exam also included an exam in adult neurology).

Yehuda specialized in neuromuscular disease while Shaul was appointed director of the pediatric department's Center for Child Development, after the previous director unexpectedly retired.

This position earned him an elegant (Southern style) office, the likes of which he would never again experience. The two families rented apartments in a gated estate of double-story homes nestled in a thick, subtropical wood home to a variety of butterflies and other fluttering beings that they had never seen before. The relaxed Southern courtesy felt like a breath of fresh air to them, after a few years in vibrant California and turbulent Israel.

All the children found their places at school. Hamutal and Osnat Shapira attended a public school and got to experience a typical American school, which included a prom to celebrate the end of the year. The girls wore smart dresses and were accompanied by elegantly dressed partners, who presented them with an impressive orchid. Itai attended a public elementary school. Dalia decided to make it easier for their kids and sent to them to a religious Jewish (Chabad) school. Tali, their oldest, was 11, and she soon rebelled, saying, "I didn't come here to learn Hebrew," and moved to a public school. Ronit, who was 10, and Gili, who was eight, stayed at the Chabad school. Shaul and Dalia soon paid the price for that decision. Ronit started saying praying every evening and questioning their Saturday trips. On school days, Gili had to wear (against his will) a skullcap and *tsitsit*, a kind of small poncho with tassels in the corners that religious Jews wear under their clothes. Luckily, as they were secular, the family stayed in Nashville for only a year.

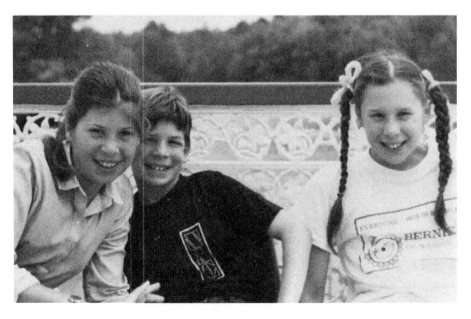

From left to right: Tal, Gil and Ronit in Tennessee—1981

Every night, the two men went to the estate's club house at the top of the hill, even on weekends when they could, and poured over the material for the exams. Despite their jobs and studies, the salaries they were earning wasn't enough for the two families to allow them to travel and have a good time, so they supplemented their income with another job—at the biggest psychiatric rehabilitation hospital in the U.S., Bottom Clover. They did alternate weekend shifts there, during which they didn't have much time to rest, as they spent most of the time in the emergency room sewing up patients who had bitten each other, cut or self-harmed themselves, or filling out endless paperwork on patients who had died.

And in between, the families found time to enjoy themselves. They traveled, mostly to the Great Smoky Mountains National Park, which was always hidden under a layer of clouds. The area boasted a few chocolate-box towns that, as one could expect, were very commercial.

A common pastime in Tennessee was a night out at country music clubs, where they played the banjo and violin quite marvelously and sang somewhat monotonous and corny songs, which Shaul found delightful and which annoyed Dalia.

Through friends they'd met in Nashville, one day they had the opportunity to meet Jimmie, Hank Snow's son, and to attend his show at the Grand Ole Opry. Hank Snow was one of the founders of country music in the U.S., and after a long and wild period of taking drugs, Jimmy became a pastor and singer. At the show, they were invited to sit on the stage, near the musicians and the charismatic singer. The hall was full to capacity, and Jimmie Snow told the excited audience the story of his deterioration, and how one day, he discovered God, or more precisely, the son of God, Jesus. And when he said passionately, "And when I saw Jesus," the crowd rose to their feet and roared like a tsunami: "Hallelujah!"

Shaul and Dalia were at a loss. They felt that rising to their feet meant accepting Jesus as their savior, and so they remained half-seated for quite some time.

257

Yes, Nashville was a deeply religious city. It had 850 churches and three synagogues that served a Jewish community comprised of only 3,000, and it was impossible not to belong to one of them. When they arrived in Nashville, Shaul and Yehuda were asked by the head of the neurology department, who happened to be Jewish, which synagogues they were going to choose. At first, out of politeness and curiosity, they chose the Reform synagogue, which he belonged to. The services were spectacular—a gospel choir was accompanied by musicians...what could be more pleasing to the ear? Although they were moved, to them it felt more like a church than a synagogue. On the other hand, the Orthodox synagogue, with all the bustle and noise, where the kids were running around and people seemed to be doing business, reminded them too much of the synagogues in Israel. Finally, they joined the Conservative synagogue, which for them had the right balance of modernity and tradition.

Shaul, who soon learned that, despite the large staff at his disposal and the splendor of his office at the Center for Child Development, they had almost no young patients, and he soon became bored. To his surprise, when he asked why, he was told that as they had to follow the strict and unforgiving rules of the insurance companies, he couldn't see the children from the downtown, public hospital at the center, which belonged to the private hospital. And it was those children who were often in desperate need of a developmental diagnosis. Also, many families in the Nashville area, which was a little behind the times, were unaware of medical services.

As a typical Israeli with a little daring, a lot of chutzpah and a great deal of good will, Shaul decided that he would fill the center with children. He contacted churches and schools, and off they went to the small towns around Nashville, between 20 and 70 miles away. Their team traveled in a short but impressive convoy of four cars and included psychologists, occupational therapists, speech therapists and physiotherapists. Whenever they passed a church or a school, they used the loudspeakers they'd rented to announce their wares like peddlers, informing the residents that they were conducting developmental screening tests for children at no charge. Anyone who wanted to have their children tested was welcome to come right away.

There was a long line in each town, and they examined them all. They then referred any child at developmental risk who they felt needed a more comprehensive neurological examination to the Child Development Center at Vanderbilt. These children, if they had any health insurance coverage at all, flocked to the center. And so, Shaul the director showed a considerable increase in the number of patients and flaunt his Israeli inventiveness.

At the end of the year, Shaul and Yehuda went to Memphis to take the first part of the board exams. Although they didn't shut their eyes all night because they were staying at a motel on a noisy freeway, and also because Shaul, with his weakness for seafood, didn't think of the risk and got food poisoning… despite it all…they passed the exams!

VIA DOLOROSA—ON THE WAY TO INSTITUTIONAL RECOGNITION OF PEDIATRIC NEUROLOGY: WHEN THE PERSONAL BECOMES POLITICAL

Upon his return to Israel, Shaul and his friends (Yehuda, Dr. Brand, Dr. Gadot and the late Dr. Weitz) continued campaigning to have the field of pediatric neurology recognized by the Ministry of Health and the Scientific Council. They wanted Israeli fellows to be able to do their fellowship in Israel and to create a curriculum of Part I and Part II exams, written and oral exams. In 1981, the pediatric neurology unit run by Shaul was recognized by the Ministry of Health, the Israeli Society of Pediatric Neurology, and by the Scientific Council. Yet, despite these recognitions and the fact that Shaul and his friends studied pediatric neurology specifically in the U.S. and were certified in it, the chair of the Scientific Council openly opposed approving pediatric neurology as a subspecialty and argued that there was only pediatrics. There was no way to overcome the barrier preventing them from achieving their goal.

Meanwhile, the group, led by Shaul, continued to lecture and perform studies, determined to persuade the new generation of young doctors to go abroad to specialize in the field, and they even helped them to get scholarships and find places to do their fellowships. They gradually began to gain recognition, if not from the academia then at least from doctors and patients, who flocked to their doors.

And one day, in the early 1990s, things changed.

One of the grandchildren of the council's chair, who was himself a well-known adult neurologist, became sick and he needed a neurological consultation. He quickly called Shaul and asked him to come to Jerusalem to examine his grandson. "I'd like your opinion," he said.

Shaul went to Jerusalem, went into the boy's room, examined him and put on a big, impressive show. He performed a differential diagnosis and explained his considerations and thoughts with the grandfather, and finally reached a final diagnosis.

He must have made a big impression, because a month later, the council chair called and asked him to do another consultation. A boy from Tel Aviv had come to his private clinic with a neurological problem, and he wanted Shaul to come with him to see the interesting case.

When they saw the boy, the council chair introduced Shaul as one of his students and then they went into another room to examine the child. Shaul was very thorough and again examined the child carefully, performed a differential diagnosis and diagnosed the problem. The two doctors went out to talk to the parents, the council chair told the parents that he'd consulted Shaul, who had studied pediatric neurology in the States, and that he completely agreed with his diagnosis.

About two weeks later, after submitting yet another of many requests for institutional recognition of their profession, and much to Shaul's surprise, the chair of the Scientific Council, who had been their greatest opponent, made a fiery speech and explained with sparkling eyes why it was so important to establish formal studies in their developing field. He went on to praise the generation of young doctors who had studied the field in the U.S. and explained how important it was to have experts in pediatric neurology. Naturally, they were given the green light that they so wanted from the Scientific Council and in 1992, pediatric neurology was recognized as a subspeciality of pediatrics.

Shaul and his friends began to take the necessary, practical steps. They wrote an official document listing the conditions that had to be met in order to establish a recognized pediatric neurology unit and answered the question of under what conditions a doctor could be recognized as a pediatric neurologist. They also prepared the written and oral board exams. In 1996, official written and oral exams in the medical specialty of pediatric neurology were held. For quite some time, 50 percent of all the pediatric neurology fellows did their fellowship with Shaul.

But Shaul's clinical success wasn't enough for him. He chose a long and difficult path and devoted part of his time to basic research, not just clinical. To do so, he worked with Prof. Ephraim Yavin from the Weizmann Institute.

In his major study on intrauterine fetal distress and brain development, Shaul contributed more than 35 articles to scientific literature, 15 chapters and countless lectures in Israel and abroad.

Because of his crucial contribution to the field, in 1988 he was made an associate professor in the research track, and a few years later, a was made a full professor. One year, the Weizmann Institute chose Shaul and Ephraim Yavin's study to demonstrate the capabilities of the Weizmann Institute.

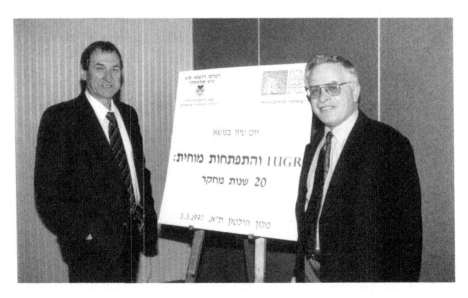

Shaul and Professor Ephraim Yavin of the Weizmann Institute

1982 - ICHILOV HOSPITAL IN TEL AVIV, ONE FIGHTER TO ANOTHER

It was his first visit to the department after completing his extra year of advanced training in Nashville. He'd been appointed head of the Pediatric Neurology Unit at the Ichilov Medical Center in Tel Aviv.

A team of doctors and nurses showed him all the babies who'd been hospitalized with various neurological problems so that they could conduct tests. He examined a few of the babies, made whatever notes, and suddenly, out of the corner of his eye, he noticed a small room that they'd left out.

"Who's in there?" he asked.

"Oh, no, forget Sima," one of the doctors responded. "She's a hopeless and tough case. Basically, she's just boarding here in the hospital. Her neurological damage is too extreme and she doesn't stand a chance."

"I still want to see her," Shaul insisted and entered the room.

Isolated, slightly apathetic and motionless, the little baby lying in the crib had a tiny body and a huge head, like an enormous, ripe watermelon.

"What's the matter with her?" Shaul asked, who didn't like giving in to the angel of death.

Two doctors answered in unison, "She has a congenital disorder of ventricular drainage and severe hydrocephalus (excess fluid) inside the brain ventricles. There is no way to help her! As her head has grown to such enormous dimensions and the cerebral cortex is very thin, the surgeons say that there is

263

no point in operating on her."

Everyone understood the meaning: severe mental damage and mortal danger.

"No one even visits her," one of the nurses added. "Her mother just abandoned her here after hearing the diagnosis and didn't want to get attached to her. She's been lying here ever since. It's been months and her head doesn't stop swelling. The doctor who's been treating her said that it's the end."

Shaul's face remained sealed. He asked the staff to let him through so that he could examine the baby. He took out the little ragdoll that he always carried in his bag and moved closer to Sima, whose fate seemed sealed.

He touched her lightly. She didn't respond. He shook her very gently and she opened her big eyes at him. He moved the doll closer to her delicate face. She stared at the doll for a long time and suddenly broke into a smile that was full of light.

Shaul's heart skipped a beat, and he felt his fighting spirit start kicking. Perhaps because he was more aware than others of the power of the spirit and of its ability to overcome any obstacle.

"Listen up," he said to the team, who was watching him intently. "If this baby, after spending so much time lying in isolation, responds with such a smile to the doll, she has vital potential. I can't give up on her, I can't leave her to die without trying everything possible."

He asked to see Sima's CT scan, immediately called the surgeon, and said to him, "I recommend that we do drainage, very slow drainage…each time, we'll carefully drain a little of the liquid out. I'm fairly sure that once the pressure is reduced, there'll be room for her brain to start developing again and grow to the necessary volume."

It took them a few weeks. Sima's brain was drained a little each time, and indeed—as Shaul had expected and hoped—once the pressure dropped, her brain slowly started to grow in volume.

And still, Sima's biological mother didn't want to take her, and she was sent to a foster family.

For ten years, Shaul kept a close eye on the girl. She grew up to be a sweet, alert child with an extraordinary sense of humor. Although she was diagnosed with ADHD and learning disabilities, she attended a regular school and did well. Her slightly enlarged head was covered with a mop of black curls. One day, Sima came for a check-up with the social worker and another woman.

Shaul asked her, "Where is your mother?"

To which she replied, "This is my mother."

And then the social worker told him that the child had received so many comments on her skin color and black curls, which were so different from her foster family's appearance, that she insisted on meeting her biological parents. Her foster family, which was loving and understanding, agreed, and when the biological mother saw how well she'd developed, she asked to take her back.

Sima's foster family was very understanding, and, in the end, she returned to her birth mother, while her foster mother became like an aunt. She was now blessed with two loving families.

Shaul was delighted to hear the news and was pleased that he'd listened to his strong intuition, despite the difficulties that the girl still had, as he was sure that she'd overcome them and be able to cope.

In 2017, Shaul received a touching phone call from Sima, who had grown into a woman. She asked if she could visit him and bring him a gift. She had found herself, at over 30 years old, feeling a need to contact the doctor who'd saved her life when she was a baby, and she asked her mother for his details.

At their moving meeting, Shaul met a sweet, confident woman who was living in a sheltered home and doing artwork.

She brought him a big, picture, wonderfully colorful, made from winding, vibrant colored paper, and on a heart-shaped piece of paper at the bottom of the picture, she wrote: "To Prof. Shaul Harel—with appreciation and thanks for the life that you granted me."

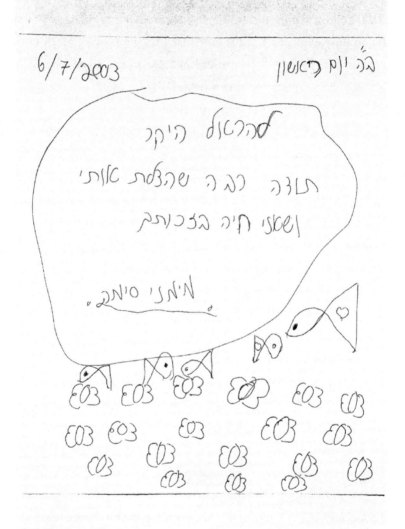

Thank you to Prof. Harel, from Sima

STAND UP FOR WHAT YOU BELIEVE IN, AGAINST ALL THE ODDS

There were a few times during Shaul's career that the medical system threw in the towel when a child received a bad prognosis, whereas Shaul never gave up.

Of all those cases, some remained engraved in his heart.

Amir was born with a severe brain defect. He was born without the corpus callosum, a part of the brain through which fibers pass from the left hemisphere to the right. That's the part of the brain responsible for the left hemisphere working in harmony with the right.

The doctors had told Amir's parents that his case was hopeless, and that he'd be mentally disabled.

When the parents, a young and intelligent couple, received the diagnosis, they cut off all ties with him and stopped visiting him in the hospital. The baby remained in the department for a few months while they tried to find him a suitable institution.

When one day, Shaul returned from a conference abroad, he quickly went to the pediatric division. Amir, who was lying there miserable and alone, caught his attention. As always, he went up to him with his famous Raggedy Ann doll and started playing with him while Shaul examined his neurological responses.

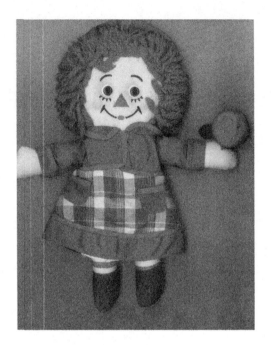

Shaul's Raggedy Ann doll

To his surprise, a big, lively grin spread over Amir's face, a smile that was on the verge of laughter. An intelligent spark flashed through his eyes. It was enough to spark Shaul's interest. He asked to see Amir's brain CT, on which the doctors had based their bad prognosis.

As he looked closely at the CT, he saw that Amir was indeed lacking part of the corpus callosum, but there were no other brain defects.

Shaul knew that medical literature indicated that most babies born without a corpus callosum also suffer from other malformations, which limit the brain from developing, but babies with a partial malformation in that part of the brain without any other malformations can develop well.

Shaul realized that this was a child who stood a chance.

There was no reason, Shaul thought angrily, *for the doctors to tell the parents what they told them.* He realized that he had to do something.

There was a soldier doing her national service at the hospital, and he told her to stay with Amir, play with him, talk to him, and not to leave him his side for a moment. And that's what she did.

The soldier spent all of her time with Amir, and he slowly started blooming. Within no time, had the entire staff captivated.

He had light hair, blue eyes and a constant smile on his lips. All the nurses in the ward fell in love with him and wanted to take him under their wing.

Shaul thought it was time to contact the boy's parents, assuming that when they saw him, they would immediately want to take him home.

When he called Amir's mother, she didn't even want to talk to him. She was afraid that he'd try to convince her to take him home. But Shaul didn't give up and he tried to reach the mother through Amir's grandmother. He managed to convince the grandmother that it was a good idea for Amir's mother to meet him. After long deliberations, Amir's mother agreed to meet Shaul but refused to see him at the hospital, so they arranged to meet at the Child Development Center.

Shaul will never forget how hard that meeting was.

Even after explaining to the family that the information they'd received was incorrect, and that he'd examined Amir, who was intelligent and functioned perfectly, his mother remained unconvinced and was still afraid of taking him home.

"Don't you believe me?" he continued. "Come with me now to the department and see for yourself."

Amir's mother looked at Shaul and said, "If you sign a document ensuring that the child will be fine and that he won't have any neurological problems, I'm prepared to take him."

Shaul looked at her in shock and replied, "My dear lady, I can't guarantee that in ten years, any child will be an outstanding student. I can promise you that his condition is now excellent, which you can see in my medical summary of his condition."

The mother refused to listen and shook her head.

Shaul's voice hardened, "I just have to explain to you," he added sternly, "that if you don't take Amir within a month, we'll have to put him up for adoption and you'll never be able to change your mind."

She didn't take her child. Shaul looked for a suitable couple to adopt him and found one.

They were both American scientists who lived in Beersheba. When they came to the hospital and saw Amir, they fell in love with him on the spot.

"Can we take him now?" they asked with sparkling eyes as they held their arms out for the sweet baby.

"No," Shaul and his staff laughed. "We have documents to fill out, bureaucracy, you know. We just wanted you to see him for the first time and to see what you think."

"We're bowled over," the nice couple said. "Can we take him already?"

From the moment go, they could both see what Amir's biological mother had refused to see. And he doubted that any other parent could have showered him with as much love over the years.

During the years that followed, Amir's parents continued to bring him to see Shaul. He grew up to be a wonderful, incredibly smart, charismatic child who spoke two languages fluently.

Some cases would touch the thin line between life and death, but Shaul learned never to lose hope.

In 2001, Shaul was asked to come to the intensive care ward at Ichilov Hospital in Tel Aviv to give a neurological consultation. They wanted him to determine the condition of a two-and-a-half-year-old toddler who had been seriously injured in a car accident and his condition was critical. They believed he may be brain dead and were considering asking his parents to donate his organs.

The toddler was lying in bed and was as pale as a sheet. His parents were waiting outside the room. Shaul looked into the mother's eyes, which were red from hours of crying, then went in to examine the child.

The determination and survival instinct that were planted in him as a child during the war and his usual use of play to examine children joined forces. He did a thorough examination, determined to turn over every stone. To his surprise, he found signs of vitality. He took his Raggedy Ann out of his doctors' bag and started to play with the boy, and after a few minutes, he noticed tiny reactions on the boy's face. Finding it hard to believe his eyes, he examined him again, but he wasn't dreaming: the boy had responded to the doll!

He ran out to inform the doctors, went to the mother and said to her, "Don't give up, your son has a chance of recovering, and he's going to live."

The boy recovered and continued with his life. Years later, the mother and her son, who was already at school, came to see Shaul and to thank him. The mother told her son who Shaul was and said, "We've come to visit your second father."

THE PRECEDENT OF THE BOY WITH CEREBRAL PALSY

Shaul's close connection with children with conditions increased his drive to make it possible for them to live a normal life and motivated him to do anything he could to help them when they grew up and wanted to enlist in the army.

Sammy, a 17-year-old teen, sat looking at Shaul with tears in his eyes.

Shaul knew Sammy well, ever since his parents had brought him to see him when he was just nine months old, and he started treating him. Half of his body was paralyzed, and he suffered from uncontrollable convulsions. Shaul continued to treat him as a boy and then as a teen, as he continued to suffer from epileptic fits, but he could be stabilized with medication. Although Sammy had cerebral palsy, he was intelligent and motivated. He studied hard and did well, despite his physical limitations.

But now, as he sat facing Shaul, he looked frustrated and unhappy. He wanted to be like everyone else. He wanted to enlist in the IDF.

"We're sorry," he was told, "the IDF can't recruit you because of your disabilities."

Sammy tried not to cry as he told Shaul, whom he so admired, what he wanted. "I want to enlist," he said. "I *have* to enlist," he repeated over and over, like a prayer. "Please help me."

Shaul looked at the determined boy with deep affection. He had a great deal of respect for the courage and determination the boy showed, but more than that, he identified deeply with him. Had he not broken through impossible barriers a few times in his life with the use of willpower alone?

"I'll help you," Shaul promised, while he had no idea if he would succeed. The challenge was complex, but he knew that he would do all that he could and fight with all of his might so that another child in the world would feel valuable; that he was on par with other children; and that in the end, it was the will and spirit that mattered.

He contacted the authorities and the IDF but was met with refusal. "He's disabled, he won't manage, it's complicated," were some of the responses that Shaul received, who didn't give up. He continued to write educated letters explaining why there was no reason not to draft the boy. But nothing helped. "We can't take the responsibility," was the final answer.

The army didn't know who it was up against. Shaul continued to insist, he repeatedly contacted the recruitment bureau, and eventually, he managed to persuade the army to recruit the driven boy.

The boy enlisted in the medical corps and came to visit Shaul in the clinic. He was wearing his IDF uniform and was in high spirits. He was so proud and happy, as if a few inches had been added to his height.

To everyone's amazement, the boy ended up being awarded recognition as the outstanding soldier of his unit.

SUDDENLY, THE FAMILY'S CONNECTION TO THE ATOMIC BOMB IS REVEALED

For years, Israel, Regina and Shaul believed that their mother's entire family—the Rotblat family—had been wiped out, except for their aunt Mira and her family, who had survived in Belgium. How great their astonishment was in the 1980s, when they learned in the most random way possible that an entire branch of the Rotblat family had made it to England when the war broke out. Prof. Joseph Rotblat was the head of the family. He was a well-known physicist from Poland, and he collaborated with the English physicists even before the war, and later helped to develop the atom bomb.

Joseph was Perla and Mira's beloved cousin, and they were very close.

Within no time, the connection between the Hilsberg and Rotblat families was reestablished, and Shaul got to know the exemplary although controversial member of his family.

Joseph was born in Warsaw in 1908 to an established and large family, and his family—like Perla and Mira's—experienced poverty following World War I. While he was studying to become a physicist, he married Tola Green, but they had no children. Whenever he visited Perla in Brussels, he spent a lot of time with mischievous little Charlie and would carry him around in his arms.

He conducted his own experiments in Warsaw on nuclear fission that scientists in England were working on and he realized the inherent potential of creating an atom bomb. He was troubled by the question of what the Nazis would do if they developed such a weapon, and he had no doubt that they would use anything, however cruel it may be, to impose their doctrine.

Since he only had minimal modern and suitable equipment at his disposal in his laboratory in Warsaw to conduct these tests, he moved to Liverpool in 1939 to join James Chadwick, who had received the Nobel Prize in Physics in 1935 and was one of Britain's top physicists. And so began the fruitful collaboration between these two scientists.

In August 1939, he received a fellowship that allowed him to bring his wife Tola to England, and he returned to Poland to bring her over. But Tola, who was recovering from appendicitis, couldn't travel yet. Due to the news blackout in Poland, none of them were aware of how grave the situation had become, so Joseph returned to England only a few days before the Germans invaded Poland. When the war broke out, he wanted to find a way to get back to Poland to get his wife out, but the British urged him to return and promised that they would not only get his wife out, but his entire family, and they would bring them all to England.

And indeed, all of Joseph's siblings and their families made it to England, but they were unable to rescue his wife Tola. All of his efforts to bring her to England through various countries, from Denmark and Belgium to the Netherlands and Italy failed and she remained trapped in Warsaw. She was sent to the Majdanek concentration camp, where she perished. Joseph never recovered from the pain of losing the love of his life, and he never remarried.

In November 1939, the brutal invasion of his country drove Joseph to suggest to Chadwick that they work together on developing the atom bomb. He was afraid that the German physicists who had remained in Nazi Germany were already doing so, and that Hitler would use it later to conquer the world.

It was a terrible time for Joseph as he faced the most difficult dilemma that a scientist can have. "I felt it's against the ideals of science to work on a bomb," he said in one interview. "On the other hand, the ideals of science were endangered if Hitler and his philosophy of Nazism were to prevail."

Joseph's contribution to developing the bomb, which he worked on with Chadwick, was significant. As he was a prominent physicist, he was chosen by Chadwick in November 1943 to join a delegation of British scientists to work in the U.S. All the scientists were required to become American citizens, but Joseph insisted on remaining a Polish citizen because he wanted to return to his country and reestablish physics research there. That was his first rebellion, but not his last. It was only thanks to Chadwick's recommendation that the Americans finally agreed to accept the proud Pole, and he was sent with everyone to Los Alamos.

The Manhattan Project was the code name for the project. Throughout that period, from November 1943 until the end of 1944, many of the scientists weighed the need to create such a deterrent against Nazi Germany against the very creation of such monstrous weapons, which were capable of bringing humanity to an end. Joseph was one of the most ambivalent of them all.

After the head of the American project told him that they were actually building the bomb to prove to the Soviet Union how powerful America was, he felt deeply betrayed. Toward the end of 1944, when Germany's defeat was certain, he thought that there was no longer a need to produce such weapons and he left the project and Los Alamos in December of that year.

The American military intelligence had a thick file on Joseph, and it contained a lot of fake evidence. He was suspected of being a communist spy, but it was agreed that he would leave, and they wouldn't reveal his "true" motives. The official reason they gave was anxiety over his wife's wellbeing in Poland. There were many differences of opinion concerning the necessity of developing and using the atom bomb. But keep in mind that in the summer of 1945, when the Americans were still wrestling with the question, the Japanese still had two million soldiers with a strong fighting spirit, and they would never have considered surrendering. They had hundreds of kamikaze pilots, young and old, who were willing to sacrifice their lives.

Joseph returned to Britain and eventually became a British citizen. He wasn't permitted to enter the U.S. until 1964. He was the only physicist who left the Manhattan Project for reasons of conscience and he slowly became one of the most prominent critics of the nuclear arms race.

Despite the Iron Curtain and the Cold War, he advocated for establishing ties between scientists from the West and East and he joined Einstein, Oppenheimer, Russell and other scientists who together founded the World Academy of Art & Science. He believed that scientists had as much moral responsibility as doctors, and that scientists, too, needed a Hippocratic Oath of their own to provide them with a code of moral conduct. He was actively opposed to the nuclear arms race and served as chairman of the Pugwash Conferences on Science and World Affairs. He and Pugwash were awarded the Nobel Peace Prize in 1995, and in his thank you speech at the prize giving ceremony, he said, "Remember your humanity, and forget the rest."

In the years that followed, Shaul's brother's family would get together with the remaining members of the Rotblat family, but Shaul met Joseph only in the 1990s, when he saw him in London. It was a very moving experience for them both. To Joseph, Shaul was still little Charlie, and it seemed like only a day had passed since he'd carried him in his arms. And Shaul had his heartbreaking story of survival and impressive medical career to share with him.

Two years later, Shaul went to visit Joseph again, this time with Dalia. It was after he had received the Nobel Peace Prize. By then Joseph was in his late eighties, a tall man with perfect posture and impressively sharp. They met at his modest home, and Shaul and Dalia had to make their way between the dozens of piles of books and booklets on the floor, as Joseph didn't have room for them on the shelves (computers were not that advanced back then). They had a fascinating talk, and Joseph stressed again that in his opinion, they should never have dropped the bombs on Hiroshima and Nagasaki, because they only did so to prove the power to the Soviet Union just how powerful the U.S. was. Others were of the opinion that they had to use the bomb to save the lives of hundreds of thousands of Americans and Japanese, and that it was the only way to get the Japanese to surrender. Joseph also solved for them the mystery of the play *Copenhagen* by Michael Frayn, which was left open ended: did the German scientist Heisenberg fail to build an atom bomb because he didn't want to take part in creating such a monstrous weapon that would be handed over to their insane ruler, or did he simply miscalculate the quantities and fail to build the bomb for technical, not moral and humane reasons?

Shaul and Joseph didn't agree on everything. Shaul didn't like his warm relationship with Yasser Arafat, especially in light of the suicide bombing attacks against Israel after the Oslo Accords. He also didn't like his enthusiastic defense of Mordechai Vanunu, whom he nominated every year for the Nobel Peace Prize. However, he did feel respect and affection for him, as he one couldn't deny his courage and devotion to world peace.

LONG-TERM RESEARCH—BECAUSE ONE SHOULD NEVER DESPAIR

During his many years of professional activity, Shaul conducted groundbreaking long-term studies related to his work with children at developmental risk. These studies are prominent in international literature. Shaul was always troubled by the question of what odds the children referred to the Child Development Center had to be a part of ordinary life, and how significant early rehabilitative and education intervention was.

The first large-scale study he did was published in 2003 and included 4,300 patients, who were tracked from birth to age five. These children were referred to the center during 1975-1994. They collected data about the families, who they were referred by and why, any social and genetic risk factors, prenatal and perinatal risk factors, as well as information on the diagnosis and treatment results.

After creating an extensive database of the various characteristics of the population referred to the center, they asked the question, which the study then tried to answer: how are these children functioning today medically, educationally and psychosocially, and how are their achievements?

This question had significant medical, educational, social and economic implications because working on rehabilitation and education and treating developmental issues early on can later lead to a marked reduction in costs and resources for the health and education systems, as well as the costs of treating and providing care for adults who find themselves being excluded from society. The results of the study were very encouraging: it turned out that most of the children referred to the center for various developmental issues became integrated into Israeli society at some point, in terms of their academic achievement and their social abilities. Awareness of the importance of early rehabilitative and educational intervention has increased over the years and has had good results. It has proved the importance of finding the rehabilitative potential of children during the first few years of their life and of helping them to recover from any damaged cognitive, linguistic and motor skills, which is possible due to the brain's plasticity and ability to change. The main message of the study was that early childhood is a critical period, during which medical, educational and welfare services should be incorporated, and that this viewpoint should consider the allocation of human and economic resources a national priority.

The results of this study, which showed that more than half of the center's patients had enlisted in the IDF (compared to 70 percent of the general population) and more than 25 percent of these served in combat units and in other key roles, convinced Shaul that the IDF's approach of automatically releasing children who were treated at the development center, thus preventing them from serving in the army, had to change. Shaul saw this as a big and unjust mistake for these children and for the army. In his meeting with the chief medical officer, Shaul showed him the research data. The boy with cerebral palsy who had enlisted thanks to Shaul's insistence and who ended up being chosen as the outstanding soldier of his unit, together with the data from the study Shaul had conducted convinced the chief medical officer. As a result, the IDF changed its approach to and procedure for recruiting people with disabilities.

At the same time as he was working on this epidemiological study, Shaul continued to work on the study he began at UCLA and then at USC in IUGR and its connection to the development of the child's brain. In L.A. he worked mainly on the live experimental model, the rabbit, which was meant to simulate human conditions. After returning to Israel, he continued to conduct (and still does) one of the largest ongoing studies in this field in the world. Over the years, IUGR and the name Shaul Harel became synonymous.

IUGR is a state of fetal distress resulting from a variety of reasons and it can occur in three to 10 percent of pregnancies. It is "responsible" for a third of low birth weights and can cause brain damage, which manifests in a number of developmental problems: motoric disorders, language problems, behavioral problems, ADHD and learning ability.

The prevalence of such cases can result from environmental conditions, such as infection, severe malnutrition, smoking, radiation or drugs—causes that are typical to people from weaker socio-economic backgrounds and occurs mainly during the first half of pregnancy. In these cases, the damage to the fetus is symmetrical (the body and head are damaged equally).

Other causes of intrauterine distress, which Shaul's study put more focus on, are high blood pressure, preeclampsia or vascular disease in the mother, which affect the second half of pregnancy. In these cases, the newborn is asymmetrical, with a shrunken body and a relatively large head (due to brain sparing, the process through which the brain is protected).

The best clinical predictor for the development of a child with IUGR was found to be the Cephalization Index, or the CI. That's the ratio between the head circumference and body weight and is based on the principle of brain sparing. It expresses the severity of the IUGR process. This index was first introduced into international literature by Shaul.

The study included aspects of basic medical sciences and was conducted in part at the Weizmann Institute in collaboration with and headed by Prof. Ephraim Yavin, the head of the neurobiology department. The staff of the Child Development Center and the Pediatric Neurology Unit were in charge of the basic medical science and the clinical part, in collaboration with Prof. Yael Leitner, Prof. Aviva Fatal, Prof. Haim Bassan, Dr. Michael Rothstein, the late social worker Ora Bichunsky, psychologists Prof. Ronny Geva, and Dr. Rina Eshel and

281

Dr. Rachel Yifat—communications experts. These dedicated research partners followed up on children exposed to intrauterine distress as a result of a restriction in blood flow through the placenta, which disrupted blood and oxygen supply to the brain of the developing fetus. The follow-up was carried out using neurological and psychological tests from the moment the intrauterine problem was diagnosed, or from the time of birth until school age, during which the children's motor, verbal, concentration and learning abilities were assessed, as well as their ability to be part of their families and of society.

The aims of the study were to identify the risk and damage factors and to neutralize them as early as possible, as well as to study the clinical indications that predict the children's functional ability at a later stage. Thus, children could be treated and rehabilitated as early possible, as there is a critical period in the development of the child's brain, from the halfway point of pregnancy until around the age of three. At this time, the brain is more flexible and although there may be irreversible damage, some damage can be prevented by detecting and treating it early.

The accepted method for diagnosing IUGR is using ultrasound and colored Doppler tests, which check blood flow in the placenta and the brain. Nowadays, even an MRI of the brain can check the size of the fetal organs, the head circumference and brain volume relative to the rest of the body. "It has been proven that when fetuses in distress are diagnosed and taken out in time, and we prevent them from remaining in poor conditions we also prevent ongoing damage to their brains," Shaul explained. In addition, preliminary findings in biochemical research have shown that the risk of restricted fetal development can be determined by taking urine and blood samples from women with high-risk pregnancies and measuring the quantitative ratio between the biochemical substance that constricts blood vessels, which aggravates the ischemic damage, and the active substance for vasodilation, which reduces the damage. A number of publications have shown that sometimes treating these conditions with aspirin results in improvement and leads to an increase in fetal weight.

Monitoring fetuses and infants who were relatively small throughout the duration of pregnancy included a breakdown of the level of risk from the parents and the environment, the pregnancy and the newborn or fetus, according to the degree of optimality. The higher the number of sub-optimal phenomena, the developmental risk to the newborn is greater. Monitoring was continued until the children were ten and included neurodevelopmental, psychological and clinical tests. The data showed that children who did not close the gap on weight, height and head circumference within the first two to three years of their lives showed higher incidence of neurological disorders (in motor coordination, graphomotor skills and spatial orientation), language quality, ADHD and learning achievements. Early detection of clinical disorders allows for earlier rehabilitative intervention during the child's development.

The study also included related projects, such as monitoring the movements of fetuses and infants of up to the age of four months by taking images of fetal movements using ultrasound and filming the infants' movements on video. These images made it possible to analyze the form, quality and quantity of the movements and to obtain important information about how the central nervous system was functioning. Findings of this innovative study, which the physiotherapist Dr. Luba Zuk participated in as part of her doctoral dissertation, pointed to the positive relationship between spontaneous motor activity of fetuses and infants to cerebral function at two years of age.

Links were also detected between children with IUGR syndrome and relatively high blood pressure, the onset of diabetes, blood clotting problems at a later age and more, in order to enable follow-up and preventive care accordingly. The link between fetal distress and sleep disorders to ADHD were also studied.

In conclusion, over the years the range of the study expanded and grew, and it provided insight into the need for follow-up and early treatment as well as for providing a good environment and early developmental stimulation for children at developmental risk who had suffered from IUGR in order to improve their functioning.

THIRTY YEARS OF RUNNING FROM PLACE TO PLACE

As mentioned, in 1981 Shaul was appointed head of the neurology unit at the Tel Aviv Medical Center and was loaned out by the unit to also run the Child Development Center, which belonged to the public health department of the Tel Aviv Municipality. The center employed about 50 personnel, from doctors to a broad team of paramedical professionals such as physiotherapists, occupational therapists, psychologists, communication clinicians, educators and social workers. The diagnostic unit and the rehabilitation units were located in different parts of the city.

Shaul was made an associate professor in 1988, and five years later he became a full professor of pediatrics at the Tel Aviv University's Sackler School of Medicine. Over the years, Shaul worked to establish the unit and he later initiated subspecialties in pediatric neurology. He sent many of his staff abroad to do specific fellowships, and thus they could establish specific services that allowed the unit to diversify its activity. Prof. Uri Kramer specialized in epilepsy, Prof. Yoram Nevo in muscle and nerve diseases, Prof. Haim Bassan specialized in fetal and neonatal diseases, and Prof. Aviva Fattal went into the field of metabolic disorders and genetics. Prof. Yael Leitner became an expert in high cognitive functions and learning disorders, and Dr. Michael Rothstein specialized in movement disorders. These were the people who developed the subspecialties they went into and who greatly promoted the reputation of the institutes called The Child Neurology Unit and the Child

Development Center. It was the first time in Israel where the work of both fields was combined. It should be noted that throughout all of Shaul's years of activity in pediatric neurology and child development, he received the support of the pediatric division director, Prof. Zvi Spirer, who always wholeheartedly encouraged Shaul's work and enabled him to develop and spread his wings.

At the beginning of his career at the hospital, while he was still developing the field of pediatric neurology, Shaul was also assisted by Dr. Uri Jurgenson, who later chose to continue into general pediatrics as Prof. Spirer's assistant, and after Prof. Spirer retired, he became the director of the pediatric division.

Since Shaul always saw the field of child development as an integral part of pediatric neurology, he was happy to take on the management of the development center (all on one salary, of course). However, the need to divide himself between different places of activity eventually claimed its price. It was hard and ineffective for him and his staff to work at three different centers, and when the Kirya Maternity Hospital and the preterm and newborn unit was active, they even found themselves running between four centers. Shaul dreamed of uniting them all both physically and from an administrative point of view.

In the first stage, he managed to move all the services from the Tel Aviv Municipality to the Ichilov Medical Center in Tel Aviv, and by so doing, the split in administrative management was eliminated. This step also allowed him to academize the institute, because by transferring it to the Ichilov Medical Center, which was of course a recognized academic medical center, the fellows could get credit for specializing in their field.

After years of running both fields, Shaul became more driven to combine child development with pediatric neurology, and he believed that the field of child development needed to be a subspecialty in pediatric neurology, just like epilepsy, metabolic diseases, neuromuscular illnesses and more. He had countless disagreements with some of his colleagues, pediatric neurologists who believed that including neurodevelopment in pediatric neurology would reduce their professional standing, which was defined as diagnosing rare and complicated diseases. Shaul, however, claimed that if neurodevelopment wasn't included, pediatric neurology would lose a broad range of treatment and a more comprehensive viewpoint that looked beyond focusing on rare diseases and syndromes. Integrating neurodevelopment in pediatric neurology would give their field prestige and raise its professional level.

At a later stage, he fought for the joint field to be recognized by the Scientific Council and for the board exams to be the same for both fields. Only after years of battle, toward the end of his career, was Shaul able to formally combine the two fields, which gave him great satisfaction. Unfortunately, the Child Development Center at the Strauss Health Center and the rehabilitation unit at Beit Abrahams moved to the Medical Center in Tel Aviv only after he retired, and he got to enjoy the joint activity site not as the director but as a professor still active in providing guidance in academic and research areas.

It should be noted that during all of his years of activity, Shaul devoted special efforts to disseminating the knowledge he and his colleagues acquired with other professionals and with the general public. This educational activity began in the late 1980s, when Shaul, together with Prof. Sydney Strauss and in collaboration with Prof. Malka Margalit and psychologist Galia Rabinovitch initiated a continuing education program at the Tel Aviv University's School of Education in interdisciplinary professional training in normal child development.

The program took place on a weekly basis and covered sensory-motor, mental, emotional, and social issues. After five years, the continuing education program was turned into a course for continuing studies at the Tel Aviv University Sackler School of Medicine and it continued for 16 consecutive years on a weekly basis. It was run by Shaul and Galia Rabinowitz.

Doctors and paramedical professionals from all fields and from all parts of the country took part in the program and it became known for its uniqueness and creativity.

At the same time, from 1996-2001, Shaul and Galia held one-day seminars and one-day continuing education programs on early childhood development on a monthly basis for professionals and the general public, with top-notch researchers and clinicians lecturing on a variety of topics, including those not included in the regular academic curriculum. These included: brain development, cognitive and emotional development, language and movement development, sleep, therapy models including play, animal therapy and contact with animals, complementary medicine, children's literature and music therapy. The course became a hit and participants came from all corners of the country, purchasing annual subscriptions.

During all these years, Shaul worked closely with a number of secretaries who were his right hand and who were of significant help in fulfilling his goals: Shoshana Rozen, who has been with him ever since she received him at the Child Development Center, and who has always been loyal and devoted; Efrat and Amit, who worked with him since they were young girls, were of great help; and Shaina Henigman, of course—the ultimate English-speaking secretary, who helped him with conferences and research papers, always meticulous and demanding, but also motherly and caring toward Shaul (despite the fact that they were of the same age).

CONFERENCES, CONFERENCES

CONFERENCES, CONFERENCES—PUTTING ISRAEL ON THE INTERNATIONAL CONFERENCE MAP

Conferences were an important component at the core of Shaul's work. Shaul was determined to put Israel on the global pediatric neurology map, and he started working on this as soon as he completed his fellowship. It wasn't only a personal ambition; he also saw it as a Zionist mission to have Israel become part of the world. He wanted Israel to draw world attention. He was convinced that one of the ways to highlight Israel's position in global pediatric neurology was to organize conferences in Israel.

After doing his fellowship in the U.S. and working on early detection of at-risk infants, he concluded that other areas pertaining to early childhood should be integrated in the field of early childhood: health, environment, education and more. In 1979, he decided that the first international conference he would initiate in Tel Aviv would be on infants at risk. His aim was to have all the top professionals from a number of fields participate. These fields included medicine, psychology, physiotherapy, occupational therapy, social work, speech and communication, education and more. The conference would result in a book summarizing the discussed topics and the conclusions they reached.

It was no easy feat. Shaul had to go abroad and personally recruit well-known speakers, such as Prof. Leo Stern—a world-renowned expert on neonates and infants, Jack P. Shonkoff—an expert in early childhood intervention,

Prof. Frankenburg—who came up with the Denver Developmental Screening Test, and others.

At first, he could only get minimal funding for the conference because it was a special initiative with a unique topic of its own. International conferences are usually held by organizations or unions who guarantee initial financing.

Shaul turned to a well-known top conference company, one of the few at the time. It wasn't easy getting the company to agree, because the odds of the conference offsetting the costs weren't high, and Shaul was relatively young and had not yet made a name for himself. When the company did eventually agree, they treated him as if he were just a marginal factor, not worth investing a lot of secretarial work in. And so, Shaul found himself spending entire evenings pasting stamps on envelopes to send to potential participants and wasting hours taking the mail to the airport (there was no internet then). Despite the many uncertainties, the conference was more successful than expected and brought many people to Israel.

When the conference was about to start, one of his secretaries came running up to him and told him excitedly that a man had proudly introduced himself to her as a communist, from some obscure place—Slovenia in Yugoslavia. And as he had no money, he couldn't pay the registration fee. At the time, Israel had no formal relationships with communist countries. Shaul rushed over to meet the mysterious man, Milivoj (Miko) Velickovic, and naturally, he waived the registration fee.

It was the beginning of a wonderful friendship and it is still going strong.

The conference broke new ground and led to a series of conferences on at-risk infants.

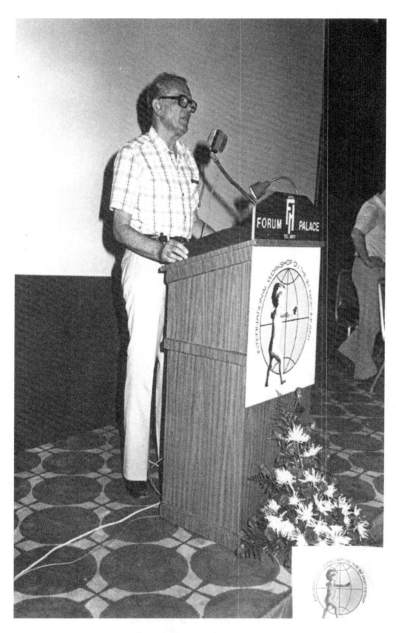

Prof. Boger addressing the conference

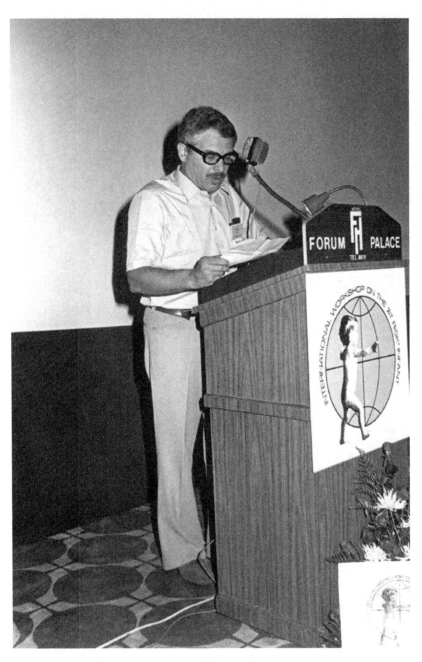

Shaul speaks at the first conference on children at developmental risk

It wasn't long before Shaul was rewarded for all his efforts in organizing conferences in Israel. Towards the end of 1985, when he was elected to serve on the board of directors of International Child Neurology Association (ICNA), and after taking a trip to Japan, he convinced them to hold an international conference in Jerusalem. It was only the fourth such conference, because the association had only been established in 1974 and was still relatively new.

In 1986, while Israel was still not as controversial a country as it is today (despite the 1982 Lebanon War), it was still perceived as a small, poor country that lacked resources and it had to compete with bigger, more developed countries.

Shaul somehow managed to convince the association's secretariat to hold the conference in tiny little Israel, despite the many conflicts in the Middle East. The conference made an impression on the participants, because it exposed them to Israel's unique spirit after less than 40 years of independence. The conference closed with an amazing performance by Kol Demama, a unique dance troupe consisting of deaf and hearing dancers.

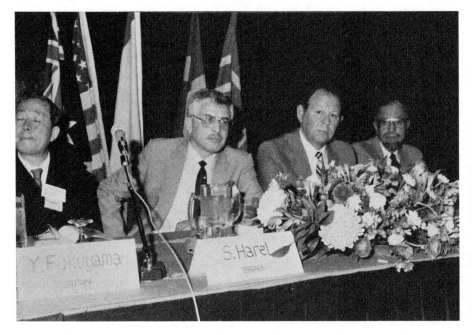

The International Conference of Pediatric Neurology in Jerusalem. Shaul, in the middle as president of the conference, and next to him on the right is Minister of Health Mota Gur

The Israelis were welcome at the American pediatric neurology conferences, but Europe was a different story. It was hard to break through the glass ceiling of the European Pediatric Neurology Society. Individuals had to be members of a regional, ethnic or linguistic sub-organization, for instance, for English, French or Spanish speakers.

Israel was controversial and didn't belong to any organization, so Israeli representatives couldn't attend European conferences as individuals. What could one do?

Shaul found a creative solution, and during the ICNA international conference in Jerusalem, he founded the Mediterranean Child Neurology Society together with the Turkish representative, Prof. Yavus Renda. The society represented all the countries in the Mediterranean, such as Cyprus, Greece,

Turkey, Italy, Spain, France and others. Over the years, the interpretation of the society's sphere expanded, and the Mediterranean joined other seas, thus adding countries such as Slovenia, Croatia and Montenegro.

The Mediterranean Society's first conference was held in Crete in 1987, followed by another 16, four of which were held in Israel. The participants enjoyed the conferences: they were held in charming locations, the program was never too overwhelming and had a strong social element, with entertainment such as tours and shows. It was an optimal combination of business and pleasure. The conferences earned a good reputation and were attended by doctors from other places, too, not only from countries belonging to the Mediterranean Society, such as the U.S., the U.K. and Russia. Many friendships were forged there.

These conferences were of particular importance at a time when Israel's political prestige was dropping, and gave them the opportunity to explain Israel's issues, whenever this was possible, of course.

After founding the Mediterranean Society, there was no longer anything standing in Israel's way and it joined the European Pediatric Neurology Society, after which Shaul was elected to its board.

In 1995, Shaul, Prof. Evrard from Belgium and Prof. Victor Dubowitz from London (one of the best neuromuscular specialists in the field) initiated a reform to the bylaws of the European society. The board decided that the society would be open to anyone to join on an individual basis, and a new European society would be established.

Shaul grabbed the opportunity and persuaded the board to have the society's first conference, in its new format, in the "very European" country of Israel, and in the "very European" city of Eilat, on the border of Egypt, Saudi Arabia and Jordan.

It was quite a battle to pull off.

The conversation went as follows:

"Do you already have funding?"

"Not yet, but I'll take care of it," Shaul replied.

"Do you have a list of potential participants?" (It was, after all, a new society.)

"No," Shaul replied, "but don't worry, we'll get it sorted."

"At which hotel will the conference be held? Does it have experience in hosting conferences?"

"Oh, the hotel is completely new. It's the most spectacular in Eilat! I admit, it doesn't have experience yet in organizing conferences, certainly not international conferences, but it's management is outstanding."

The members of the board were stunned by Shaul's answers, but he was so self-confident that he convinced them, and they agreed to have him organize the conference at the Royal Beach Hotel in Eilat.

Prof. Victor Dubowitz, the president of the European society and of the first conference, wrote about it in his memoir, noting that "that's what you call Israeli chutzpah."

Shaul set his creative imagination free at the conference. One afternoon, they went sailing in the Red Sea on an armada of boats, from which they all jumped into the sea. After that, they had a hearty barbecue prepared by the hotel staff. On another day, Shaul arranged a tour of the mines in Timna Valley. Of all the events, the gala evening was firmly engraved in all of their memories. They were taken by bus to a mysterious spot in the Eilat Mountains and dropped off into the pitch darkness. The lights immediately came on, and against the backdrop of the mountains, they saw a sensual belly dancer moving to the sounds of music. They were served an impressive spread in a huge Bedouin tent, where everyone sat cross-legged on carpets and cushions. The next thing they saw was a camel train carrying the world's top pediatric neurologists dressed in colorful galabias, who then gave a passionate recital of the pediatric neurologists' ten commandments when finding themselves in the middle of the desert.

The evening ended with a fun disco party in the heart of the desert—a very unusual phenomenon in the history of formal European conferences.

That was the conference that put Israel on the world conference map.

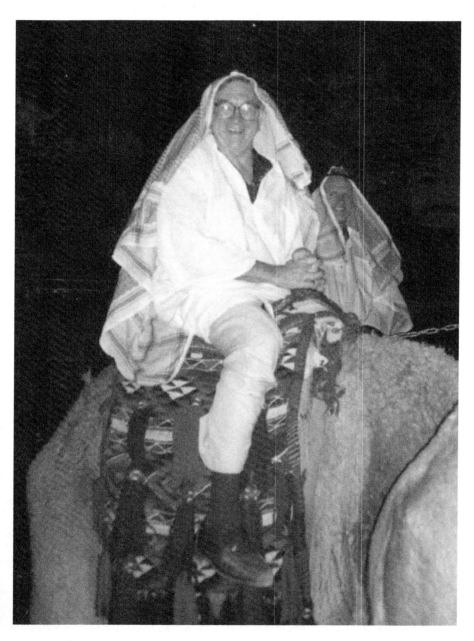

Prof. Dubowitz, President of the European Pediatric Neurology Society (EPNS)

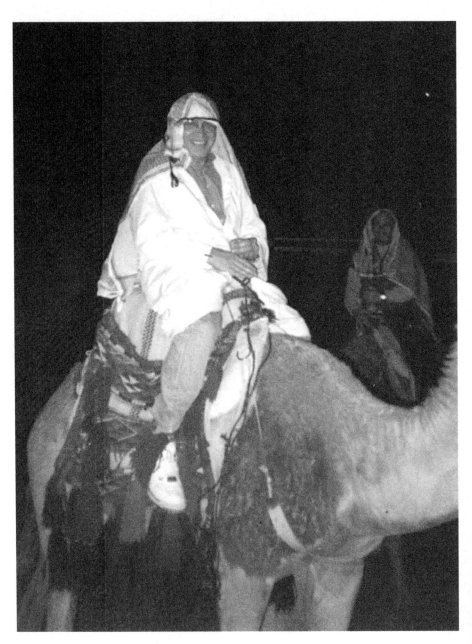

Shaul, president of the conference

Another series of conferences included the joint conferences held for the two disciplines of pediatric neurology and pediatric neurosurgery. There had long been the feeling that there was a lack of serious discourse between the two disciplines, which treat the same children but don't read the same literature and don't participate in the same conferences. The time had therefore come for each to learn about the research and practices of the other.

The initiative for collaboration between the two fields came from Shaul and Prof. Fred Epstein, a senior neurosurgeon in the U.S., who treated mainly children. Shaul and Prof. Epstein met in 1988 and over the years, their friendship grew deeper and made an impact on Shaul. Fred was extremely professional and humane by nature. He was modest but charismatic and he offered help to anyone who needed it. He had extraordinary medical skills, and he was also very Zionistic and a big supporter of Israel.

Shaul and Fred decided that the conferences would be called New Horizons in Pediatric Neurology and Neurosurgery and the first conference was to take place in Tel Aviv in 1990.

It was through Fred that Shaul met Shlomi Constantini, his outstanding student, with whom Shaul later established the joint neurology and pediatric neurology clinic. The clinic was unique even on an international level and was a true benefit to the children and their families.

Prof. Epstein's wonderful career was cut short by a terrible drop of the sword. In 2003, when he was riding his bike through his neighborhood, he fell into a pit that hadn't been marked with any hazard signs. His brain stem was severely injured, and after being unconscious for two months, the doctors recommended to his wife to disconnect him from the machines. She refused to throw in the towel. Against all the odds, he got back on his feet, but he couldn't continue working as a surgeon.

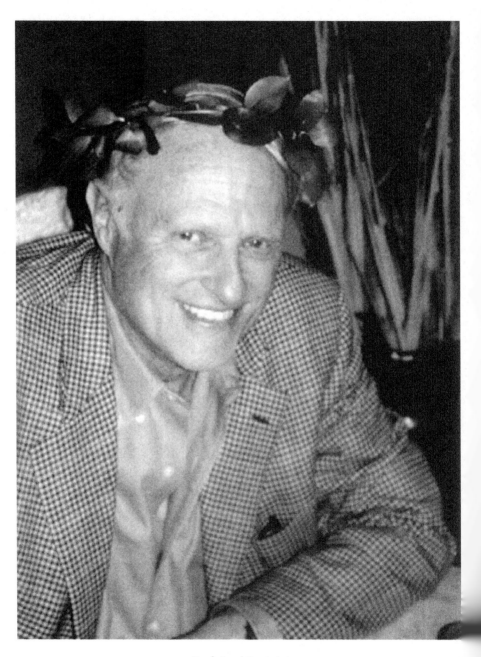

Prof. Fred Epstein

Shaul was disappointed by the American medical establishment's attitude toward Fred following the accident. From being an invincible celebrated surgeon who founded special departments at both the NYU and Beth Israel hospitals, which were world renowned, Fred became disabled, lost his livelihood, and was barely assigned a small office after he returned to the hospital.

In 2005, after he'd recovered, he attended the third New Horizons conference and was treated with honor and respect. He surprised the participants with his eloquent speech and vision, and it was decided that from then on, the conferences would be named after him. Sadly, he never made it to another conference because fate had other ideas. A year later, he died suddenly from melanoma. He was not yet 70 years old.

Two conferences in his honor were held after that. Fred's story illustrated to Shaul how fragile people are, how fleeting their glory and status.

Due to all his work, Shaul was elected to serve in several international positions. He was a member of the International Child Neurology Association, or the ICNA, and he served as the association's secretary from 1998-1994. In 1998, he was elected president of ICNA at a conference in Ljubljana, Slovenia, and he served in this capacity until 2002. He saw this as an achievement for Israel.

As president of the association, he set up the ICNA education committee, with the aim of promoting a number of courses in pediatric neurology and child development, especially in developing countries. He was also a member of the secretariat and was active in the European society for many years.

Over the years, Shaul organized about 20 international conferences and was a driving force in assimilating Israel in international activities. It wasn't easy. He was always afraid that there'd be a suicide attack that would result in a high number of victims, or of a minor war that would prevent participants from abroad from attending. But Shaul, who was known for his tenacity and perseverance, didn't give up, as he saw the conferences as a means of creating a bridge between Israel and other countries. To his delight, luck was on his side and they never had to cancel a conference.

A symposium that missed the bullet by a hairline was held in the fall of 2000 and marked the new millennium. It was held at the Notre Dame of Jerusalem Center in the auditorium that Pope John Paul II had inaugurated that March. It was a spontaneous conference that Shaul initiated after his friend Franco Guzzetta from Italy invited him to attend a conference in Assisi. It was being held by the Vatican to mark the new millennium, and would be attended by the three main Abrahamic religions. The topic of the conference was "Birth: the Beginning of Developmental Freedom," and it would include an ethical discussion of fetal rights from the viewpoint of the three religions.

When Shaul received the invitation, he immediately called Franco and suggested, "Why not start the millennium with a symposium in Jerusalem, since it's holy to all three religions, and then we'll continue in Italy?"

Franco, a devout Catholic, had strong ties with the Vatican and he passed the proposal on to senior officials there.

The Vatican eagerly accepted the proposal and made one request: to hold the symposium at the Notre Dame of Jerusalem Center. To Shaul's surprise, Monsignor Luizzi, the pope's academic secretary and the Vatican's representative, was a tough negotiator by all accounts, despite the Vatican's phenomenal wealth, which shed a light on why the Vatican was so financially successful.

The Vatican wanted them to hold a commemorative concert in the John Paul II Auditorium at the center, with representatives from the three religions. There wasn't much time to organize it, about a month-and-a-half, and Shaul asked his friend the musician Hannah Levy. Within no time, she arranged a rich program with volunteer performances by mixed Jewish, Muslim and Christian orchestras and choirs, and by performers such as David Daor, Shlomo Gronich and the Sheba Choir.

The concert was moderated by the Vatican's ambassador to Israel, Archbishop Pietro Sambi, an impressive man with whom Shaul developed a friendly relationship. The atmosphere was wonderful and the audience in the hall included not only professionals from abroad and from Israel, but also Christian clergy, Muslim qadis and Jewish rabbis. The Vatican's ambassador to Israel spoke and said, "When I see all the dignitaries of the three religions sitting here together, sharing in this solemn concert, my heart expands with joy."

It was only a few weeks before the second intifada broke out and took everyone by surprise. No one expected it to continue for years and claim many lives on both sides.

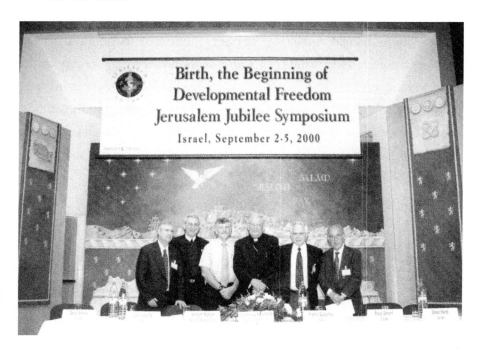

The conference at the Notre Dame of Jerusalem Center. Shaul is second from the right, next to the Apostolic Nuncio to Israel

The discourse on fetal rights continued in Italy, starting in Assisi and ending in Rome, with Pope John Paul II attending. The participants in the final symposium received a commemorative booklet, the title of which was *From Jerusalem via Assisi to Rome, making* Israel's part in the significant event clear.

The closing ceremony for all the symposiums sponsored by the Vatican was held in the Vatican's main hall and was attended by the pope, respected clergy and 5,000 participants. Enthusiastic speeches were made, and the choir (conducted by a well-known Jewish conductor) sang heavenly hymns. Shaul and Dalia sat in one of the front rows and couldn't help but be impressed by the beautiful, majestic ceremonies

At the end of the event, contributors to the event were invited up to the stage to receive the Pope's blessing. Only 50 people were given this honor. Monsignor Luizzi started calling people up to the stage. He was delighted when he noticed Shaul, and he invited him to come up. Shaul and Dalia could feel the envious glances from their Catholic friends. Those called up to the stage were received with the angelic voices of the choir. When Shaul went up, he naturally didn't kiss the pope's hand like the others, but he did bow and shake the pope's hand before saying, "I'd like to take this opportunity to express my appreciation of the Christians who put themselves in danger, hid me and saved me during World War II."

As the pope was already suffering from advanced Parkinson's disease, Shaul found it hard to detect his response, but he felt that he had now had closure, and Dalia, who held Christianity accountable and felt resistant, had tears in her eyes despite herself.

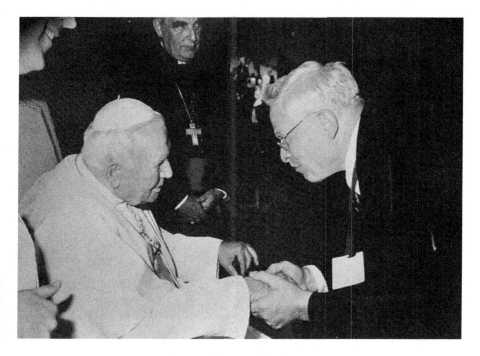

Shaul with Pope John Paul II

This was not the only time that Shaul met a pope. A few years later, Shaul was invited to another symposium at the Vatican, and again, Monsignor Luizzi noticed him and asked him to come up to the stage to receive the blessing, this time by Pope Benedict XVI. And again, all of Shaul's Catholic friends wondered how Shaul, being Jewish, was receiving such an honor, and for the second time, too. Naturally, all encounters between the Pope and people from the audience was photographed and then purchased for a fitting sum. When Shaul received his photo, he was surprised to see that (perhaps accidentally) his hand had cupped the pope's, instead of the pope holding his, or as his friend Victor Dubowitz wrote jokingly when he shared the picture with others: "When Shaul Harel blessed the pope."

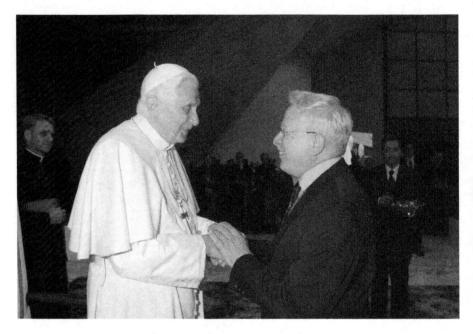

Shaul with Pope Benedict XVI

It wasn't the first symposiums where Shaul felt closure in his life. In 1995, 25 years after the Child Development Center was founded and Shaul was the director, he felt that he had to mark the significant date. He gave a lot of thought to the performance that would mark the event, especially as he didn't have adequate funding.

When he was already on the verge of despair, he had a chance professional meeting with the head of Tel Aviv University's Research Authority, who surprised him with a proposal—to organize a cantorial music event, something that Shaul was far from an expert on (even though his father was an amateur cantor).

The head of the Research Authority was himself an amateur cantor and assured Shaul that he would help him along. They contacted the head cantor of the Great Synagogue of Jerusalem, Naftali Hershtik, and with his help, the best cantors in the world volunteered to perform at the event.

Shaul arranged for the cantors to visit Beit Abrahams to witness the rehabilitation work they did with children with disabilities, and they promised to honor the amazing work with their marvelous singing. The management of the Medical Center in Tel Aviv weren't sure that the event would be a success, but it was, and a great one at that. Cantorial enthusiasts such as Mayor Shlomo Lahat of Tel Aviv, Jacob Frenkel, the Governor of the Bank of Israel and others were more than happy to attend.

Shaul opened the event with a speech, in which he mentioned his only memory of his father, wrapped in his tallit in the small shtiebel, or synagogue, just down the road from home, and that for him, the event was also in memory of his father.

The guest cantors and the boys' choir sang wonderfully, the psalms touched everyone's heart, and the performance received rave reviews in the press.

Shaul's colleagues were very appreciative of Shaul's extensive activities in their professional field and in organizing international symposiums. They also knew his life story and were amazed by his resilience and relentless motivation to advance and prove himself.

In March 2009, the 4th Fred J. Epstein International Symposium on New Horizons in Pediatric Neurology, Neurosurgery and Neurofibromatosis was held in Eilat. It was about a year-and-a-half after Shaul retired from the pediatric neurology unit and the Child Development Center.

Five of his friends spoke touchingly in his honor: Prof. Paul Rosman of Boston, Prof. David Stumpf of Chicago, Prof. Victor Dubowitz from London, Prof. Philippe Evrard of Paris, and Prof. Milivoj (Miko) Velickovic of Ljubljana. Shaul's sister Regina also attended. She was very emotional and had tears in her eyes, and although she had to use a walker, it didn't stop her from joining in the Israeli folk dancing, with Miko, an old family friend, as her dancing partner.

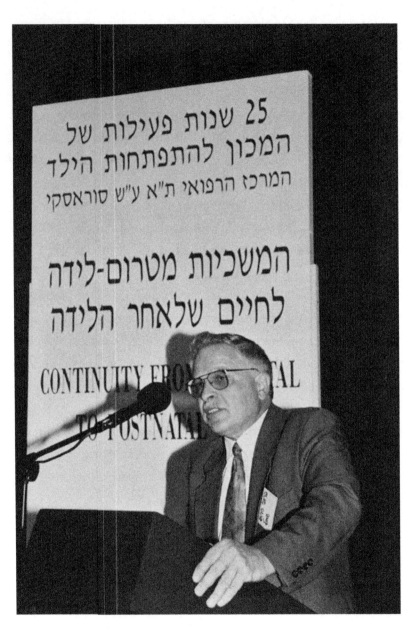

The Child Development Center celebrates 25 years

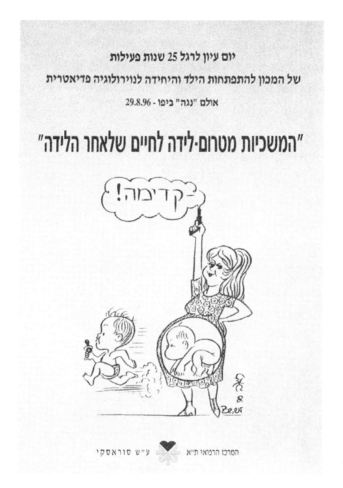

Conference: Continuity from prenatal to post-natal life

Shaul was moved not only by his peers' show of appreciation but also by the reactions he received from students and interns at the lectures he gave abroad.

In October 2000, Shaul was asked to give a guest lecture on his research at the Children's National Hospital in Washington. He was introduced at length by Roger Packer, Senior Vice President of the Center for Neuroscience and Behavioral Medicine at the hospital, who talked about Shaul's personal history during the Holocaust. After the talk, a resident by the name of Dr. Elizabeth

311

Prazza came up to him with tears in her eyes and handed him a short poem that she'd written when she heard his story and lecture. She said, "I was very impressed with your lecture, but mostly, I was moved by your story, and I couldn't stop myself from writing this poem as I listened to the lecture.

A time long ago—a child
Frail—near death
Saved by others through compassion
Fast forward to today—a child
Now an expert in fetal development
Who was to know the many lives saved
In saving this child
I am sitting in this lecture hall
Observing a miracle
Thank God for the miracle

PARTICIPATING IN CONFERENCES—WHEN HISTORY CHANGES BEFORE YOUR EYES

As Shaul also had an academic career, he would attend international conferences both to stay up to date, but also to attract conferences to Israel. After all, in the 1970s, keeping informed via electronic means was not yet an option. Even at the beginning of their careers, as young fellows in the U.S., Shaul and his friend Yehuda attended the first conferences at which the American Child Neurology Society and the International Child Neurology Association were founded. It wasn't easy for them to finance because they didn't have the means, and they had to sleep at sleezy and cheap hotels. On occasion, a drunk would sometimes come knocking at their door, and the only weapons they had at their disposal were umbrellas.

The nature of the conferences changed according to the place where they were held. The American conferences were held annually and offered a great deal of content, with an emphasis on research topics. They included an early morning seminar, which required the participants to get up at the crack of dawn. From a social and entertainment point of view, they were boring. In contrast, Shaul found the European conferences very engaging, because they dealt not only with research but also with clinical topics, and they also offered social and cultural programs.

Still, Shaul found the Mediterranean society's conferences the most enjoyable, with their perfect balance between social entertainment and professional interest.

Apart from keeping up to date professionally, Shaul (and sometimes Dalia) also got to see the events and historical changes that were happening, mainly in the communist bloc countries in the late twentieth century and the beginning of the current century, first and foremost, in Slovenia.

Slovenia. Shaul became more familiar with Slovenia in 1984, thanks to his friendship with Miko Velickovic, who invited him to visit when Slovenia was still part of communist Yugoslavia. There were no signs yet of its dissolution or of the ruthless civil wars it would experience later, in the early 1990s.

The standard of living in Slovenia was low, the hotels were government-owned and the meager food they offered was served to the table by grouchy women.

A few years later, Slovenia would be the first to battle for and demand its independence. Shaul and Dalia kept track of the events, concerned for their Slovenian friends, Miko and his wife Tatiana, who managed to sneak out and make it to the symposium in Tel Aviv. Slovenia was lucky to gain its independence within a week and with almost no losses. But within no time, ruthless civil wars broke out between Serbia and Croatia, between Serbia and Bosnia and Kosovo, wars that caused terrible damage to these countries, the signs of which are still evident today.

Only in 1988, Shaul returned to Ljubljana, Slovenia, for the International Child Neurology Association's conference. The country already looked completely different, quite Western, and was starting to resemble its neighbor Austria.

It was at this conference that Shaul was elected president of the ICNA, a title he was proud of mainly because it was so significant for Israel. As usual, Miko, the president of the conference, went out of his way. After the election results were final, he marched solemnly out of the hall with the previous president, Prof. Suzuki from Japan, on one side and Shaul on the other, like a bride and groom being led down the aisle with the famous wedding march by Mendelssohn playing. In one corner, there was a huge wedding cake in their honor, which was sliced and served to all the participants.

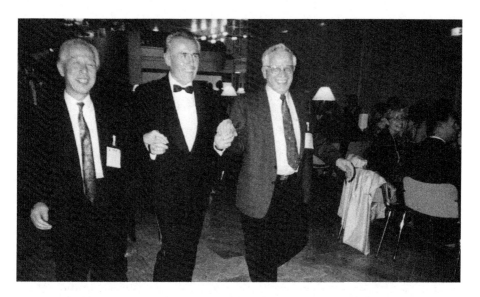

Shaul elected president of the International Child Neurology Association

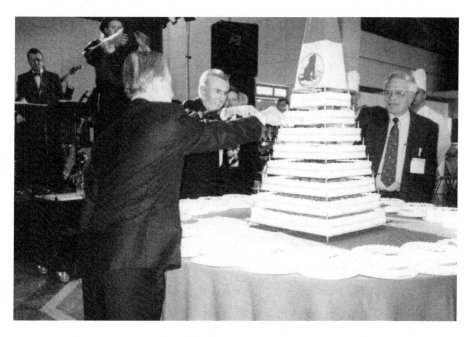

The Election Cake

In the 1980s and early 1990s, the failures and weaknesses of the communist regime had become clearer in other countries, too, such as the Czech Republic, Hungary, and, of course, Russia. The close link between the status of senior doctors and their ties with the Communist Party was blatantly obvious, and it didn't always match the level of their professional skills.

At a European conference held in Prague in 1989, Shaul and his friends were astonished when they saw the local conference organizer's magnificent home, even if he was now the head of a hospital department (a political appointment). Being a senior figure in the party, however, is what really determined his status. His house had a swimming pool, the kitchen was lined with Swedish teak, and was more luxurious than any of his foreign guests' apartments or houses. It also stood in stark contrast to the wretched housing estates they passed on their way to Prague. However, as was common at the time, the organizer was shameless and didn't shy away from doing the rounds at the conference trying to sell his worthless Czech cash to the conference guests for British pounds or American dollars.

In contrast, his colleague, who had a lower administrative position and rank, and was held in great professional esteem by his Western colleagues, lived in a shabby apartment on a neglected street in Prague. Years later, after the Czech government was replaced, Shaul learned that the wealthy doctor-organizer who had been so well connected, had disappeared altogether form the Czech medical map, and perhaps even from the country.

In 1989, Prague was incredibly beautiful but sad and somber. Teenagers strumming guitars could be seen here and there, their faces serious. There were almost no cafes or restaurants, and when Shaul and his friends wanted to go to the famous pub *The Good Soldier Svejk* at nine forty-five in the evening, the chairs were already piled on the tables and they were told sourly that the pub closed at ten. On Shaul's next visit to Prague, in 2005, after the city had already become a central tourist attraction in Europe, they could barely make their way to the famous sites, and the restaurants were open until the middle of the night.

In Budapest, too, it was important for doctors to have ties with the Communist Party, whether direct or indirect. While the person with the greatest professional authority in pediatric neurology in Hungary (who was probably not affiliated with the party) lived in a modest apartment that was barely big enough for his needs, his student, who was married to an important theater director, who was a communist activist, lived in a spacious and elegant apartment.

In regimes such as those, everyone did their best to survive, and everyone knew instinctively that when they asked a question or booked a table at a well-known restaurant or café, it was always a good idea to give a small tip, or in other words, a bribe.

Some of these things changed after the regime changed and communism fell, but it's interesting that many of Shaul's doctor friends from the communist bloc, perhaps because they were older, felt that their status as doctors had fallen along with the regime.

Of all the conferences that Shaul attended, his visit to Russia in 1992 was the most unforgettable. This time, the conference began in Kazan in Tatarstan, and continued on an Austrian ship with a trip down the Volga to Moscow. It was an unforgettable visit.

Over the years, Shaul had made friends with people from all over the world, and one of these was Prof. Badalyan from Moscow, who attended almost all of the pediatric neurology conferences in Europe. Prof. Badalyan, a tall man, looked quite the character with a white mane and an impressive deep voice. He was of Armenian descent and always pointed out to Shaul how much the Jews and Armenians had in common. He was never without cans of fine caviar and bottles of good vodka, and during conferences, he and a few of his colleagues would abandon their wives to spend many an evening in his room until the small hours of the night. Despite his poor English, he was considered one of the best neurologists in Russia, and he was a member of the Scientific Council. Only a few doctors were given that honor. He always arrived at conferences accompanied by an impressively large man who would always be introduced as a cultural attaché, but everyone knew he was a kind of bodyguard.

Shaul was actually invited to Kazan by another colleague, a Jewish doctor by the name of Prof. Ratner, after he did a study with a German doctor and discovered that the main cause of most neurological diseases and neurodevelopmental damage in children was the traumatic birth method, which caused brain and neck damage. They developed a treatment method that focused on the lower part of the skull. Ratner had the support of Sergei, one of the new tycoons that had sprouted up in Russia, a former KGB man in Tatarstan, who had taken over part of the health insurance in Russia and envisioned an international treatment center that would make a fortune treating hundreds of patients a year (similar to the Pető method developed in Hungary that was adopted in Israel).

Ratner invited 25 peers from Europe, including Shaul from Israel, to hear about their theory and to gain their support. When Badalyan learned that Shaul was attending the conference, he urged him to visit on the way and be his guest in Moscow.

Changes were on the horizon in Russia, it was after Gorbachev's perestroika and Shaul and Dalia weren't sure it was a good time to visit. The signs of change were clear: trying to replace the centralized Soviet system that had failed with a more liberal system of supply and demand, which was predicated on capitalism, all the controls and regulations had been abolished, and the economy had basically collapsed. Shaul and Dalia could see the challenges during their visit.

Prof. Badalyan gave them a warm welcome when he came to pick them up in his battered Cadillac, testimony to better days. Before taking them to the place he'd insisted on arranging for them to stay instead of at a hotel, he surprised them and took them to a concert in a magnificent hall. The atmosphere in the hall was electric, and even though it was the middle of the afternoon, the audience was dressed in their finest clothes. At the end of the show, everyone rushed to the stage holding red lilies to express their appreciation to the performers, a Russian custom that Shaul and Dalia had never seen before.

But after the impressive concert came the fall. Dalia and Shaul would be staying at a guest house for parents of children with mental disabilities. The building was gray and dirty and there was an old woman holding a bunch of keys sitting on each floor. Their room was small and long, with two narrow single beds with thin mattresses, and the toilet had no seat. In the fridge, there were sweet Bourekas, a chunk of Kashkaval cheese and mugs with black coffee. In the morning, they each received two slices of dark rye bread and a hard-boiled egg. Only later, when they saw the almost empty government stores that lacked even staple products, Shaul and Dalia realized and appreciated the efforts being made to feed them.

Some stores had pyramids of one type of canned goods, from seaweed and sauerkraut to canned tomatoes. They learned that food was being rationed for the first time since World War II.

Although the Western media was taken with Gorbachev's charisma and praised him for the fall of the Berlin Wall, people in Russia were hungry. The dinner at Prof. Badalyan must have cost him his monthly salary, but it was still meager, with green onions served as a course. The change in Badalyan's status, after belonging to the elite, had carved furrows in his forehead and face, and he suddenly looked old. When a police officer stopped him in the street and tried to extort money from him, under a false pretext that it was the only way police officers could make a living, Dalia and Shaul heard him repeatedly say, "I'm an academic, an academic." This appeased the police officer, who took pity on the doctor and made do with a hug and a small bill. Despite his dire situation, Badalyan insisted on paying for them wherever they went. He arranged tours for them to all the tourist attractions in Moscow and even bought their train tickets from Moscow to Kazan, an eight-hour trip on a rickety old train.

The poverty in Kazan was similar. All the guests at the conference were led to an old-fashioned building that had served as a sanatorium and made the convalescence homes in Israel in the 1950s look magnificent in comparison. Dalia and Shaul didn't have an in-suite bathroom and had to share with another couple, and the shower was no more than a water pipe connected to a faucet. Although the sanatorium was on the banks of the Volga, it was hard to see the river through the thick swarms of mosquitos. And the battle against those mosquitos turned out to be the biggest challenge of the conference.

Early every morning, a bus would arrive to pick up the guests, including their spouses, because there was no food available at the sanatorium or in the vicinity and they, too, needed to be fed.

At the conference, Ratner's theory was torn to shreds by the other participants, and Sergei the tycoon's face went sallow. The catering operation was impressive. Twice a day, at lunch and dinner time, the guests were escorted to a restaurant by a convoy of motorbikes (for protection). The restaurant was quite fancy compared to the rundown neighborhood, and there, amazingly, they were served hearty meals, all at Sergei's expense.

Around the restaurant there was an army of hungry-looking people hoping for leftovers or even for a whiff of food, which made the guests a little uncomfortable.

The food was quite tasty, but the chefs sometimes found the raw materials challenging to work with. They did all that they could, and when they managed to get their hands on a piece of meat from some poor skinny cow, they would cut the steak as thin as possible. Even then, Dalia's fork bent when she prodded the steak. It was anyone's guess if it was the steak or the fork at fault. Dalia believed it was the fork, further proof of the communist regime's failure. The communists had invested in producing advanced weapon systems but couldn't produce decent consumer goods. She took the fork home to Israel, proving that Russia was nothing more than a paper tiger.

In the evening, the guests were invited to attend a concert at a stunning hall. One of the best baritones in the world was performing. They thoroughly enjoyed it. There was just one thing that bothered the overseas guests, and that was the disparity between the grandeur hall and clothes that the audience was wearing, the abundance of lilies showered on the performer, and the terrible state the public toilets were in. It wouldn't be mentioned here had it not been for the shocking absence of doors to provide privacy, the lack of toilet seats, paper (even newspaper), the horrific filth and the stench hanging in the air. This image characterized every public place they visited, from fancy concert halls and restaurants to hospitals (which naturally should be sterile). Did this stem from a basic disregard for dignity and wellbeing that characterized the communist regime? In any case, more than 20 years later, when Dalia and Shaul visited St. Petersburg, they were delighted by the sparkling clean bathrooms in the restaurants, and they saw this as proof that Russia had changed.

After Kazan, the conference continued on a magnificent Austrian ship that Sergei the tycoon chartered. The cruise from Kazan to Moscow took a few days and passed through picturesque towns dotted with the onion domes of the Russian Orthodox churches. They held lectures in the mornings and had an excellent live band playing in the evenings that got them all dancing. Although there was famine in Russia, they were served five meals a day and had an unlimited bar at their disposal, again, all at Sergei's expense.

Shaul became very friendly with Sergei, who was looking for contacts in Israel to pave the way for him to do business with investors from the U.S. Shaul, who couldn't hold his liquor, found himself dancing the kozachok with Sergei as everyone clapped along. When Shaul returned to Israel, he called a well-known insurance agent and told him about Sergei. The insurance agent found out that Sergei was an infamous Russian mafia man, and Shaul would be well advised to keep his distance.

Prof. Badalyan passed away two years later, as did Prof. Ratner, who organized the conference in Kazan. They were both relatively young. Dalia and Shaul thought that perhaps the deterioration in Badalyan's standard of living and drop in status broke his heart and contributed to the deterioration in his health, whereas when it came to Prof. Ratner, they wondered if Sergei had had him eliminated after his vision of an international center to treat brain-neck damage didn't materialize.

The unforgettable trip to Russia ended in St. Petersburg (which had been called Leningrad until the year before their visit, a signal of Russia's attempt for cultural change). A year before that, a couple of Russians had attended a conference that Shaul organized. One of them was a Jewish man from St. Petersburg who was in charge of the laboratories and medical equipment purchasing at the largest neurosurgical hospital in Russia. The other was the head of the hospital. At the request of the Jewish doctor's Israeli relative, they waived the conference registration fee because of the tough financial situation the Russians were in. Neither of the doctors attended the lectures but they were more than happy to participate in the social events. They promised Shaul that they'd reciprocate when he came to Russia. Dalia and Shaul didn't pin much hope on their promises, but they really wanted to visit St. Petersburg.

To their surprise, the head of the laboratories was waiting for them at the train station with a large, modern SUV and he took them straight to a fancy, western-looking hotel. He gave them a tour guide for two days and insisted on covering all the expenses. He told them that after the fall of communism, his financial situation improved drastically, and he now had hundreds of thousands of dollars in a foreign bank. He no longer planned to emigrate to Israel. Although he was still responsible for purchasing medical equipment for the hospital, he now represented huge medical equipment suppliers and saw no conflict of interest, because the hospital chief always made the final decisions. They barely saw the hospital chief because he was about to leave for a conference, naturally somewhere exotic and at the expense of one of the suppliers. While many Russians had to spend hours trying to obtain basic food, fuel or other commodities, the man responsible for purchasing medical equipment had several servants to do that for him. A number of times, Shaul and Dalia saw cars pulling off the road into a side alley to buy stolen fuel from a fuel tanker at an exorbitant price.

It was 1992 and Dalia and Shaul got to see the beginnings of chaos, corruption and the exclusion of entire communities from the most basic level of existence, a phenomenon that they witnessed again in 2013 when they returned to St. Petersburg. This time, these were hidden behind renovations, better maintenance, tycoons with luxury palaces, elegant brands in the stores, and beautiful escort girls in fancy restaurants that only few could afford to eat in.

In 1990, Dalia and Shaul and a few of their Israeli friends visited China. They needed visas and were under constant surveillance. They had a government-appointed guide, and their schedule was also dictated to them. Tourism to China from Israel had just begun. Before that, they attended an international pediatric neurology symposium in Japan, where they received a lavish welcome in the best of Japanese etiquette, including a Noh show and a traditional tea ceremony, which was held in the hosts' tiny houses. They were showered with gifts and felt that the Japanese people had gone out of their way to impress their guests. Japan then was one of the most advanced countries in the world

They knew that China lagged far behind Japan, but they were intrigued by the country with the largest population in the world, an ancient culture and a bloody history, both because of the cruel oppression of Mao Zedong, which lasted for decades and resulted in the death of tens of millions of Chinese. The cultural revolution, the events of Tiananmen Square in 1989, and other, later events all made Dalia and Shaul very curious.

Although the reform initiated by China's new leader Deng Xiaoping had already begun with Chinese-style socialism, the standard of life in China in 1990 was still extremely low in comparison with Japan.

At the rather gray airport, they were greeted by a guide who spent the entire seven days by their side, never leaving them except in the evening, when they would relax at the hotel bar. The splendor of the hotels stunned them, especially the attractive elevator girls on each floor, with a long slit in their dresses.

The guide decided where they would eat, and to their disappointment, the food in the crowded, shabby local restaurants were no match for the excellent food at Chinese restaurants in the West. It was also hard to find food without shrimp or pork, and some of their friends, who kept kosher, had a problem. At a certain point, after they kept on returning their meals to the kitchen, they were relieved to be served what they believed to be pigeon thighs. Dalia and Shaul realized from the taste that they were frogs' legs. Since their kosher friends were already devouring their meals, they didn't dare to tell them.

Shanghai was the first place they visited, and when they walked around the Bund, the legendary waterfront, they were pinched by the locals who couldn't believe that the strange creatures they were seeing were human, and they received countless requests for photographs with the locals. It was strange to feel like creatures from outer space.

Shanghai was still a long way from its later and more modern character. There were still none of the skyscrapers that later competed with those in Manhattan and Hong Kong, and the most elegant streets were those with luxury hotels built by prosperous Iraqi Jews in the 1930s.

The waterfront was dull and neglected, people were still dressed in Mao suits, and they were surprised to see slits in the small children's pants, which served as an opening for them to go about their business and to save on diapers.

Their schedule was very strict. They were taken to a public school to watch a musical performance and rhythmic gymnastics display. They marveled at the rigid discipline and uniform movements.

Beijing was still dull and plain looking, but they caught a glimpse of magnificent houses behind walls, which belonged to party members.

The Great Wall of China had not yet been made more accessible, there was no cable car yet and the stairs were difficult to climb. There were dozens of shabby stalls with peddlers selling souvenirs. The streets of Beijing were used mainly by thousands of bicycles, big trucks and just a few fancy cars belonging to party members. They were still relatively empty without traffic jams and the air was clean.

Every hospital they visited had traditional medical departments where children walked around with needles sticking out of their faces and huge black pots of strange smelling herbs were boiling in the kitchens. There were huge piles of cabbage leaves drying in the yards. The highlight of the trip came after a few days of tasteless food, when the guide received permission from some mysterious entity to take them to a "charming" restaurant, where they could finally have a hamburger and fries with a regular lettuce salad on the side. It was the most delicious meal they ate in China.

In late 2002, when Shaul was the president of the International Child Neurology Association, he was again invited to China to open and conduct another international conference. It was hard to believe that 12 years had passed since their first visit.

Beijing had completely changed. They were preparing for the Olympics and there were construction sites everywhere. The noise of hammers and pickaxes began at five and lasted until eight at night. Whole neighborhoods were flattened and replaced with large buildings. The Great Wall of China was now accessible by cable car and tidy stores had replaced the stalls. The historical sites now had organized entrances and spotless toilets that even had soft background music playing. Shanghai was now more impressive than Hong Kong and could give Manhattan a run for its money. At night it looked more like Las Vegas, with its bountiful colorful lights. The streets were wider and had several lanes, but with that, the number of cars on the road had grown at an incredible rate, and the air was now heavy with smog.

The hospitals that the Israeli delegation visited were smart, shiny and organized. Appointments with doctors and treatments were orderly and surpassed those in Israel. The varied food (except for fried shark skin, which for some reason was considered a delicacy) tasted more like the Western world's version of Chinese food and the restaurants were huge and spacious. Just the rickshaw they took through the hutongs was reminiscent of old China. All the development had occurred in just 12 years and China's history changed rapidly right before their eyes. It was clear that it's power would only grow.

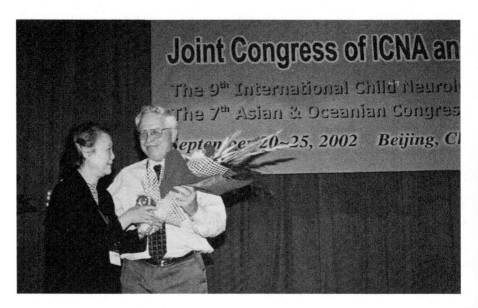

Shaul, when president of the association, at an international conference
in China in 2002

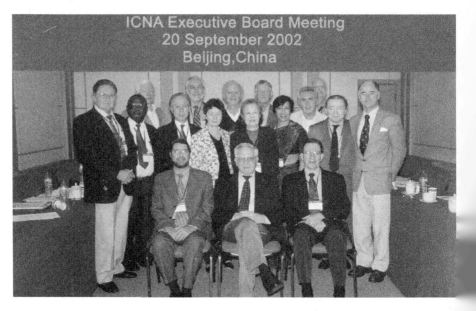

Shaul with the International Child Neurology Association (ICNA) board of directors

I HAVE A DREAM

Although his brother and father perished as a result of medical experiments, and despite the fact that many doctors in Germany (more than their relative percentage of the population) took an active part in the Nazis' atrocities, Shaul still believed that medicine could pave the way for hostile populations to connect. During all his years working at the Tel Aviv Medical Center, he treated Arab children from Gaza and the West Bank, and he saw medicine as a bridge to peace. He liked to quote one of the fathers from Gaza. The man had a number of children with epilepsy, who were treated at the neurological clinic at Dana-Dwek Children's Hospital. "I assure you that none of my children will ever throw a stone at a Jewish soldier," the man said to Shaul.

After the Oslo Accords were signed, and despite the suicide bombings within the Green Line that took the Israelis by surprise, it seemed that they could still create a database to be used for collaboration in the medical field.

At one of the social events that Shaul participated in, for Israelis and Palestinians, he met Dr. Hatem Abu Ghazaleh, a doctor from Gaza, who left a strong impression on him. He came from an old and affluent family and graduated from Oxford University's medical school. His English was perfect, he was a true intellectual, and he amused them all with stories from his student days. Hatem and Shaul clicked instantly.

Hatem had to come to Israel three times a week for dialysis, and because of his illness, he changed his specialty from surgery to rehabilitation of children with disabilities. He was the president of The Gaza Center for Cultural and Service Development. Shaul and Hatem clicked immediately. It was at the beginning of Ehud Barak's term as prime minister, traveling between Gaza and Israel was relatively easy, and Shaul even went to visit Hatem at his elegant home.

Even before that, with the hope for peace in the air, Shaul dreamed of establishing the Israeli-International Pediatric Neuroscience Institute. Together with his colleague, Prof. Shlomi Constantini, the head of the pediatric neurosurgery department at the Tel Aviv Sourasky Medical Center, he submitted a detailed plan for the center, specifying the medical and clinical services it would provide to children from the region and to the institutions they would collaborate with. The clinical services would include child development, pediatric neurology and neurosurgery, neurological rehabilitation and specific educational services. The program would offer courses in coaching and education for experts in Israel and the countries of the region, initiate national and international conferences and publish current professional literature. They also planned research opportunities. Shaul was aware that there was no such center in the region and that the level of care provided to children with special needs in other countries in the region was even worse than in Israel. It should be noted that their attitude toward the other countries was not paternalistic or arrogant, but rather expressed a desire to collaborate and help to establish similar services in the region. Shaul ended the proposal with the following words: "I believe that a project of this kind will bring us all welfare and pride and will make a modest contribution to the construction of a bridge to peace in the region."

To provide all these services, a building of about 54,000 square feet was designed by an architect that would be built near the Dana-Dwek Children's Hospital. In 1999, the plan received the warm blessing of Prof. Gaby Barabash, the director of the Tel Aviv Medical Center. After Shaul showed the plan to Hatem, the two of them concluded that they should plan a sister center in Gaza at the same time. They submitted a joint plan, signed by Shaul, Prof.

Shlomi Constantini and Dr. Hatem Abu Ghazaleh.

Shaul worked hard to make the project a reality.

On February 13, 1999, the Palestinian Authority's Minister of Health, Dr. Riyad Zanoun, sent the following letter:

"On behalf of the Palestinian National Authority, I would like to extend my support to the proposed regional cooperation project between the Gaza Center for Cultural and Service Development and the Institute for Child Development and Pediatric Neurology, Tel Aviv Sourasky Medical Center and Tel Aviv University.

It is hoped that if this cooperation project materializes, a Palestinian pediatric, neurology and neurosurgery center will be founded in Gaza as a sister to the center in Tel Aviv University. As part of this project, comprehensive child development and rehabilitation services will be created in the Gaza Strip. The creation of the above-mentioned services will be a major boost to meeting the needs of infants, the new born, and other children in the Gaza Strip, the West Bank and beyond. I encourage donors to seriously consider and allocate the funding needed for bringing about the realization of this fine project."

The letter continues with praise for Dr. Hatem Abu Ghazaleh's work in developing services for infants and young children, including a home-based early intervention program. It goes on to describe Hatem's instrumental part in providing university training programs in Gaza as external campuses to the University of Calgary in Canada, and Lamar University in Texas and Marquette University in Wisconsin in the U.S.

It should be noted that Hatem requested that the project in Gaza be a non-governmental organization so that no "commissions" would be charged along the way and all the money they raised would serve only the project.

Now it was time to start raising funds. A few months passed and Shaul contacted the Foreign Ministry. David Levy was the foreign minister in Ehud Barak's government, and he'd been invited to sign an agreement in support of the regional peace plan. Switzerland was responsible for regional collaborations, and the joint Palestinian-Israeli project of establishing the two centers was included in this category. They still had a long but promising way to go before the project could be realized.

Along the way, however, there were disappointments, some even ridiculous.

As president of the International Child Neurology Association, Shaul wanted to promote training in pediatric neurology and development for pediatricians in the Palestinian Authority, even before the project was established, which he was certain would take years.

He enlisted the help of the association's secretary, Prof. David Stumpf. He contacted the head of the pediatric ward at the children's hospital in Gaza, whom he'd met at a number of conferences abroad. He asked her to arrange a meeting with representatives of the pediatricians and community doctors in Gaza and the West Bank, which she did. The topic of the meeting was: producing a regional comprehensive course to which they'd attract the best lecturers in the field from all over the world. The course had to be held in Gaza, including a lecture hall, technical equipment and living arrangements for guest lecturers and participants from overseas and from the West Bank. Funding was to come from the International Child Neurology Association. But the results of the meeting were disappointing and Shaul and David returned to Israel empty-handed and despondent.

First, it turned out that there was no medical representative from the West Bank. Second, the doctors from Gaza were vehemently opposed to conducting a large-scale course within Gaza. They were only interested in receiving scholarships for advanced training programs in Western countries. To Shaul and David's surprise, they also refused to include doctors from the West Bank in these scholarships. When Shaul and David asked, in any case, to see the hall they

330

were planning to use, they discovered that their hosts didn't even have the key.

It was on that harsh and symbolic note that the meeting ended. David Stumpf, who was always diplomatic, couldn't help but remark, "You'll need a lot more patience to achieve collaboration in the region."

Ironically, they had a hard time getting out of Gaza, not because of the Palestinian border guards, who were gracious, but because of an Israeli soldier who was still wet behind the ears and not very smart. David Stumpf didn't have the right exit document, and after hours of waiting, Dalia, who worked for the Ministry of Agriculture, came to their rescue and called the Directorate of Agriculture Coordination and Liaison for help.

All their dreams were shattered when the second intifada broke out in October 2000 and all ties were severed. There was no more talk of regional collaborations, especially after Hamas came into power in the Gaza Strip in 2006.

Shaul tried with no success to find out what happened to the Abu Ghazaleh family. All that he could do was continue to provide care for hundreds of children a year from the West Bank and Gaza at his clinics, with permission from the Israeli Security Agency, better known as the Shin Bet, and to invite doctors from the West Bank and Gaza to the international conferences he organized in Israel.

Shaul wondered if he would ever get to see any form of collaboration in a joint Palestinian-Israeli project to treat children.

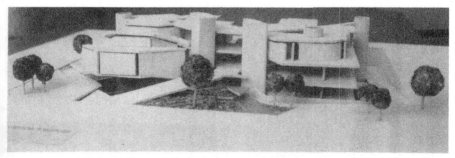

SCHEMATIC MODEL
● THE ISRAELI-INTERNATIONAL PEDIATRIC NEUROSCIENCE INSTITUTE ●

ACHIEVEMENTS AND HONORS

As mentioned, Shaul had the honor of being one of the founders of pediatric neurology in Israel, when this field was almost non-existent until the first fellows returned from the U.S. and began the struggle to develop it and have it recognized as a field in its own right. Undoubtedly, Shaul's determination and tenacity stood out, and he was a driving force in this regard. At the request of the Tel Aviv Medical Center's management, Shaul continued as Chief of the Pediatric Neurology Unit and the Child Development Center until mid-2007, when he turned 70.

In 2001, Shaul received the Ministry of Health Award for Excellence and Contribution to Medicine. In 2010, he received an award from the Child Development Society for his lifetime achievement and contribution to the advancement of child development.

מדינת ישראל
משרד הבריאות

פרס מנכ"ל
לשנת התשנ"ט 1999

מוענק

לפרופ' **הראל שאול**

מהמרכז הרפואי "סוראסקי", ת"א

כאות הוקרה והערכה
על תרומה ועשייה מיוחדת
לקידום ושיפור השירות

ד"ר בעז לב
המנהל הכללי

ירושלים, התשס"א 2001

Award from the Director General of the Ministry of Health

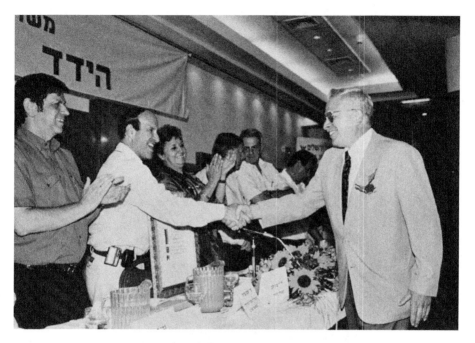

Ministry of Health Award for Excellence and Contribution to Medicine

In 2011, he received an award from the Mediterranean Child Neurology Society for excellence and contribution to the advancement of the association.

And then, in October 2011, he was invited to Savannah, Georgia, to receive the Arnold P. Gold Foundation Humanism in Medicine Award from the American Child Neurology Society. His devoted student, Dr. Haim Bassan, decided that he was worthy of this recognition and nominated him. Shaul won and went to Savannah with Dalia, his son Gil, his daughter-in-law Hila, and his little grandson Ofir. Gil and his family were living in the U.S.

Prof. Rust of Charlottesburg, Virginia, wrote a poster describing his many career accomplishments, which was displayed at the entrance to the hall.

Prof. Paul Rosman of Boston delivered a moving speech in Shaul's honor, and spoke about Shaul's extensive work and humanity. Needless to say, Shaul was very moved and after the speech, he responded in a strangled voice, "If only my parents could have been here to see me." And although he was usually restrained and in control, he couldn't stop his tears.

Everyone in the hall rose to their feet and gave him a long round of applause. Many of the guests told him afterward, "We aren't sure that we'll remember the conference, with all its presentations and lectures, but we won't forget your response to the prize."

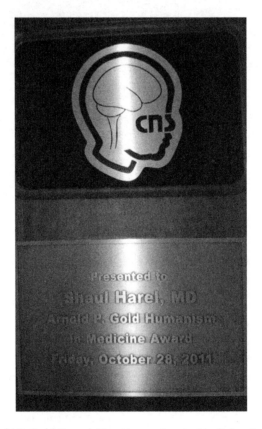

Arnold P. Gold Foundation Humanism in Medicine Award

Still, Shaul considered his family to be his greatest achievement. In less than four years, Dalia and Shaul changed from a couple with the threat of infertility hanging over their heads to a tightknit and close family of five, with three young children. Whenever Shaul came home from a hard day's work, he would hear his children and their friends cheering and playing, and his heart would swell. The Harel home was known in the neighborhood and youth movement to be welcoming, and the children's friends loved coming over. The commotion never bothered Dalia or Shaul.

When they could afford to, Dalia and Shaul always took their children abroad with them, and sometimes their grandmother Yehudit would also join them. They always said that they invested in experiences, not in assets.

Tali, who was exempt from compulsory army duty because of the surgery she had, volunteered and served for two years in the navy. Ronit was a shooting instructor, while Gili served as a tank commander, and then as an officer.

Later, they each found a field that they found interesting and challenging. Tali specialized in languages and like her father, fell in love with French. After living in Paris for a few years and completing her academic degrees, she began to work as a translator.

Ronit also obtained a master's degree and worked as an organizational consultant.

Gili completed his master's degree in business administration, and specialized in hospitality at Cornell University, which has an excellent program. After graduating, he began working in the high-tech aspect of the field. After many years in the U.S., Gili and his family returned to Israel and he continued to manage high-tech and tourism projects.

And then, of course, there are the grandchildren—Idan, Noya, Inbar, Ofir, Ido, Liam and Mia. They light up Dalia and Shaul's life, and the close bond that the children and grandchildren share.

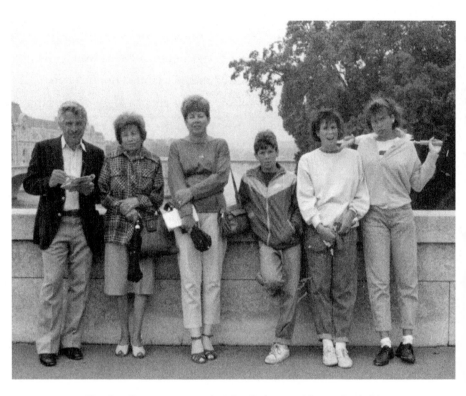

The family on a trip with Yehudit (second from the left)

BREAKING THE PACT OF SILENCE AND COMMEMORATIVE ACTIVITY

BREAKING THE PACT OF SILENCE/THE SHADOW OF MEMORY

The neurological explanation for memory loss resulting from trauma is related to the secretion of stress hormones (cortisol and adrenaline) at a time of emergency. The role of these hormones is to prepare the body to cope (the flight-or-fight response). A high dose of cortisol stops the activity of the hippocampus (where explicit memories are stored) but it increases the activity of the amygdala (where implicit memories are stored, including emotional memories). This means that severe stress can stop the explicit, conscious memory from working, while the implicit memory stores the emotional responses. This can cause a person not to remember the trauma itself, but to remember well the emotions it came with, such as fear and sadness.

When does that moment arrive, when you can trust yourself to recall traumatic memories without being overwhelmed or falling apart? For some people, that moment never arrives.

Shaul felt confident enough 60 years after the traumas he experienced and decided to remember. He made a conscious decision, after years of silence; of silencing himself both inward and outward.

"My father wraps me in his prayer shawl and I listen to him singing in the synagogue...my parents disappear...a strange house...a cold woman who makes me work hard...I'm hungry...Nazi soldiers playfully lifting me up onto their knees...another woman, plump, scrubbing her husband's scrawny back

341

in the small tub…the war is over…my brother Israel comes to visit me in hospital…a convent, a white night shirt…a large courtyard with a tree in the center…Siegi Hirsch—and laughter again."

These flashes appeared in no particular order. They were the first images to reappear in Shaul's memory, and it wasn't easy. For 60 years, his memory had been enveloped in the protective shadows of repression. Without those shadows, he probably wouldn't have been able to continue, but they also blurred and masked his ability to reexperience his memories in a new context, and thus, to have the relief of confession. But when the moment to remember arrived, it took tremendous effort to pull back the curtains and look through the window at the memories of his past. And not because he was afraid of looking into the past, as that fear had almost dissipated. He had just become used to not remembering. He was like a person who for decades chooses to sit in a wheelchair and whose leg muscles have degenerated. The person decides to stand but fails at first and is forced to proceed slowly and carefully.

His memories were buried under thick, stifling layers, and like old furniture stored in a dark warehouse, the dust was impossible to remove. Perhaps it could be done under hypnosis, by taking the bypass to the unconscious.

But the will is stronger than any mechanism. Shaul decided to look directly into the past and at the child he once was. Like a fighter before an important battle, he prepared his heart and his mind for whatever his encrypted memory would dig up. He was ready to return to the sights, the feelings and sensations, the sounds and the fears, and also to the joyful moments at the end of the war. Because, among other things, he had to answer an important question for himself: what was it that motivated him to survive those days with such bravery, to bury any reminder of self-pity, and to fight to reach that moment in 1998, when he became the president of the International Child Neurology Association?

BACK TO THE PAST

One miraculous and unexpected day, the past decided to knock on the door to Shaul's mind. He was driving home in the evening, and while he was changing the radio station, he suddenly heard the most heavenly cantor music he had ever heard. A clear, delightfully emotional tenor voice was singing, and it sent inexplicable shivers down Shaul's spine. The radio presenter introduced the singer, Joseph Schmidt, one of the greatest opera singers from the 1930s. He was born in Romania, he studied in Berlin, and at one point was even popular with Goebbels. Being short in stature, he had appeared on stage in only one opera, *The Troubadour*, in Belgium. In 1942, he perished in a refugee camp in Switzerland as a result of medical neglect. Something inside Shaul was shaken. *Who is this singer*, he asked himself, *and why does his voice penetrate my heart like that?*

Shaul had a feeling that he'd heard that voice before, and he started to look into Joseph Schmidt's life story. As if obsessed, he looked for every rare recording and every movie that Schmidt appeared in. He spent evenings at home listening to recordings of Schmidt singing. This, while knowing nothing about how their lives had once been intertwined. When the Tel Aviv Municipality named an alley by the Opera House after him, Shaul attended the ceremony as if he were a lost family member. How surprised he was, then, when he brought his brother a set of Schmidt CDs and learned that not only was he one of his father's favorites, but that he had also visited their home in Brussels in 1938.

He had run his hand over baby Shaul's light curls and fallen in love with his older sister, Tola.

That was the first time that Shaul felt any longing to connect to his past. Was it the hand of fate guiding Shaul, after 60 years of silence, to listen to the powerful and pure voice? To start exploring what he'd chosen to forget?

Two years later, at an Industrial-Commercial Club gathering, when his friend Amir Makov introduced him to everyone and mentioned what he'd been through during the Holocaust, one of the members urged him to give his testimony at Yad Vashem. At first Shaul was hesitant, but because he felt bad refusing, he went to Beit Wolyn, Yad Vashem's Givatayim branch to give his testimony

The experience shook Shaul to the core, and he found it hard to watch the video recording they gave him, because it was there that he cried for the first time.

However, the first significant encounter with his past dramatically changed his attitude to his experiences during the Holocaust. It was in 2003, when he was 66 years old. That was when he visited Auschwitz after the conference he was attending in Warsaw. Over the years, he'd had plenty of opportunities to visit Auschwitz, but he had chosen not to. It was on this visit that he first discovered how his brother was murdered in medical experiments performed by Prof. Johann Paul Kremer and that his father had died in his clinic from "exhaustion." He was shocked and felt guilty for not researching his past before (he had been to Brussels many times without bothering to go see where he had lived with his parents); for always being very nonchalant whenever he spoke about what he'd been through during the war, sharing funny episodes from his time in hiding, like the tram driver's back being scrubbed by his wife Lucy; for saying nonchalantly, "As a child I had to make do with potato peels, so I'm crazy about mashed potatoes with butter."

Shaul slowly began to delve into his past, knowing that with every memory he activated (such as the location where the repressed experience occurred)

he would evoke another memory. But the repressed memories started to become clearer, like a painting with edges that are still hazy and out of focus. The images were partial, and the missing bits were filled in by talking to others who'd been there.

His brave and beloved sister Regina, who was always there for him, and who he would care for later like a father for his daughter, filled in the missing and hazy pieces of the puzzle. Slowly but surely, he collected the missing slivers of memories into fragments of information, and he tried to knit the old fragments together by meeting up with people who had been there with him, some of whom he saw as the ghosts of his childhood.

In 2004, about a year after visiting Auschwitz, he attended a secretariat meeting of the International Child Neurology Association in Brussels, and finally decided to visit his childhood home.

"By no means can you go alone," his good friend David Stumpf, the society's secretary said. David knew a little about Shaul's life and he asked to come with him, knowing that it would be an emotional visit. Shaul was very moved by his American friend's offer and they headed off to the Saint Gilles district where he'd grown up. The neighborhood had changed and most of the residents were now of Arab descent, from Morocco and Algiers. They went to 37a Montenegro Street, where he'd lived with his family in 1937-1943. That was the place where it had all ended so cruelly, but not at all, surprisingly.

When he got there, he was amazed to see that the building hadn't changed, and the front door still had the same handle. First, he tried to find people with a Belgian-sounding surname, as they may have been able to remember his family. When he did, he introduced himself and told them that he'd lived there as a child in the late 1930s and early 1940s and asked to come in. To his disappointment, he received a firm no. In the end, out of desperation, he rang the home of an Arab by the name of Abu Khalipha, who was kind and cooperative. The man was originally from Algiers, a lawyer who fled for his life from the religious fanatics in Algeria. He now owned the building and he let Shaul into the apartment on the right side of the second floor, their apartment according to Regina.

The apartment looked like it had been frozen in time since 1943. Excited, Shaul rang Regina and described all the details to her, which she eagerly confirmed: the long corridor, with the bedroom leading off, the living room that had also served as another bedroom, with an exit to the balcony, where Shaul's bed was, the small kitchen at the rear, overlooking the yard, the kitchen cabinet that they stored the Passover dishes in. Shaul asked the Abu Khalipha to see the wall at the top of the stairwell, behind which he had hidden with his family, but he didn't really understand what he meant. Shaul, his friend, and the owner climbed the dozens of exhausting stairs up to the attic, where the storerooms used to be, including Shaul's father's. The rooms had been converted into small apartments. The wall was there, and it now served as the exterior wall of the top floor tenants' shower stalls. And then Shaul started remembering one of the most terrifying moments engraved in his mind in 1943…of standing tremoring on the top floor with his mother, who was muttering the Shema Yisrael prayer…of his father with Regina…a rag stuffed into his mouth, while on the other side of the thin wall, a German soldier stood smoking a cigarette, being too lazy to take one more step and unwittingly saving their lives.

For Shaul, it was not just a visual memory, but also of a voice screaming. That voice sometimes pierced his mind in the night. It was the scream of his Jewish neighbor who lived on the first floor as she clung desperately to her husband being dragged away by the Nazis. She was dragged down the stairs with him and she was in the advanced stages of pregnancy by then, with four other children.

Shaul and Abu Khalipha parted warmly, and he promised to allow Shaul into the apartment when he came to visit again.

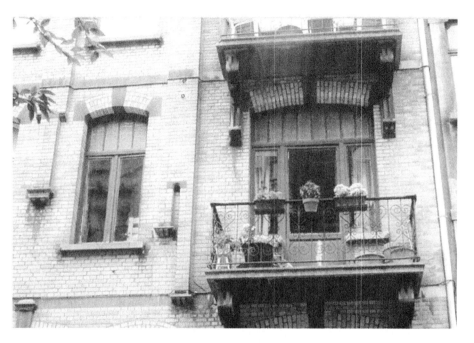

The apartment at 37a Montenegro Street

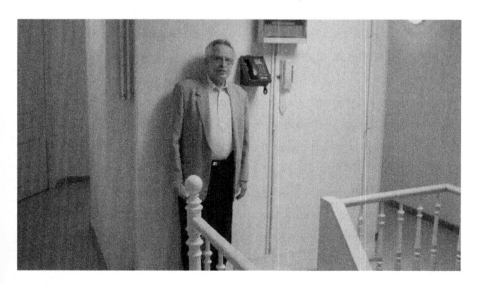

Shaul by the wall that saved him

In the summer of 2005, Shaul went to visit Brussels again, this time with Dalia, and Regina and her family. This was Regina's first time back in Belgium, in fact, it was her first time abroad in 42 years. She was already 77 and found it hard to walk. She had to use a walker and sometimes a wheelchair, which they took with just in case. This didn't stop her from enjoying life, and her mind and sense of humor were stronger than ever.

The night before they left, she could barely sleep, she was so excited. The first place they went, of course, was the apartment on Montenegro Street. The tenant wasn't there this time, but they received a warm welcome from the Algerian owner. Regina swept her hand over ever spot in the apartment; here, in the living room was where Charlie's bed stood, or should she say Chierkele, as they called him in Yiddish, because he was like a little duster sweeping across over the floor. His bed was right by their parents. They, too, slept in the living room. Here was their father's workshop, leading from the living room, where he manufactured ties with the help of their older brother, Israel. Their oldest sister, Tola, lived in the middle room. She was stunning and looked a lot like Hedy Lamarr. And despite the nine-year age difference between them, she and Regina were good friends and would whisper secretively to each other at night. There was a small room at the end of the long apartment that Israel and Marcel, their middle brother, shared….and there, in the middle of the apartment, was the kitchen. It was small but warm, and it could contain the entire family of seven. When Regina saw the cabinet where their mother stored the Passover dishes, she burst out crying. She remembered the ceremony of changing the dishes over before Passover began.

On their way downstairs, Regina pointed out the apartment where the Czechoslovakian butcher and his family lived, and she told Shaul how the Germans took him away from his pregnant wife and their four children. Shaul remembered with a shudder the screams of the woman that had been with him for years. He was swamped by a memory of playing with those children, downstairs in the hallway leading from the building entrance to the stairwell.

Despite finding it hard to walk, Regina made it up the 66 stairs to the top, where she stood facing the wall that had saved them from immediate danger.

Before leaving, Regina gave the owner a hug and said, "Fate led you, such a kind man, to be the owner of this building, and by so doing, has enabled me to visit our apartment again."

Later, the family visited the orphanage in Lasne, where Shaul first lived after the war. Shaul had difficulty finding the place. They asked around and were sent to the son of the man who was the mayor during the war and who'd taken over from his father. The ex-mayor gave them a warm welcome. He knew what they were looking for, and they managed to find the orphanage with his help. The building had changed slightly over the years and had been turned into medical clinics. It was still picturesque and surrounded by the big meadow with the stream trickling softly by. No wonder Shaul remembered the place as a small paradise.

The ex-mayor told them a story, which described how courageous many Belgians had been during the war. With the consent of the Germans, they had housed Jewish orphans whose parents had been sent to extermination camps at the orphanage. Not wanting to divulge the secret genocide, the Germans told them that the adults had been sent to labor camps. The orphanage, with the counselors who had to wear a yellow badge, was supposedly sponsored by Dowager Queen Elisabeth, but like a number of other institutes, it was being used as a stockpile for whenever they needed to fill up the carriages on transportations to Auschwitz. The Germans planned to send all the children and their counselors to Auschwitz when the time was right.

One day, toward the end of the war, the Germans decide to put their diabolical plan into action. Somehow, the Belgian underground heard about it and told the townspeople. They immediately took the children and their counselors from the orphanage and hid them wherever they could, in and out of town. They hid them in basements, barns, churches - you name it. They worked wonderfully together and none of the children were caught by the Germans.

349

Shaul and his family were very moved by the story.

The visit to Belgium was marked by Regina's 77th birthday, which they celebrated in an excellent fish restaurant overlooking the harbor in Antwerp. Regina was over the moon and reminisced about that trip for years.

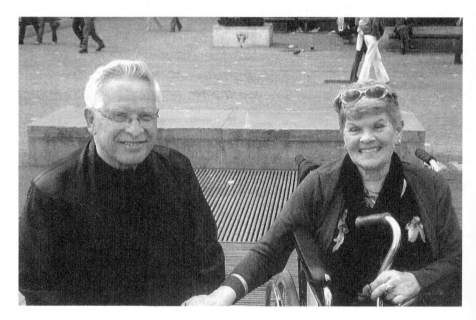

Shaul and Regina in Brussels, 2005

AND THE JOURNEY CONTINUES

From that point on, Shaul's trip back in time rapidly gathered speed.

In August 2006, Dalia and Shaul met Andree Geulen, who as mentioned, was one of the pillars of the operation to rescue Jewish children in Belgium. She was 85 years old, but no one could call her old. She stood tall and straight, her blue eyes shining from her beautiful face, and her mind and memory were as sharp as ever.

It was when visiting her at home that Shaul found the document reporting his transfer on February 17, 1943 to the orphanage, and the document for the family health services, which included his secret code, 0423. His name had been changed to Charles Van Bergen. Regina was renamed Helen. Together, they looked at the famous notebooks that the Jewish rescue organization kept and listened to Andree recounting fascinating stories about the wonderful resistance movement. Andree was still an inspiration to everyone around her. She radiated vitality, curiosity and humane empathy, just like she always had. She devoured every bite and every drop of wine at the neighborhood restaurant, claiming that water was only for **external use.**

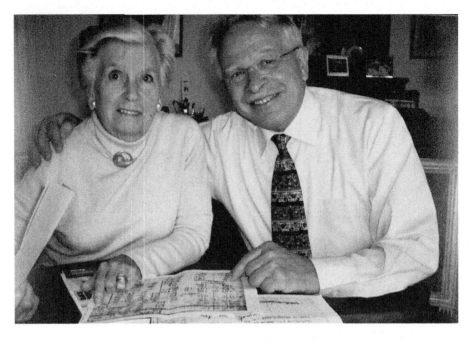

Shaul with Andree Geulen in 2009

Later, Dalia and Shaul went with their Belgian friends, David Inowlocki and
Robert Fuks, who had also been hidden as children, to see Shaul's first hiding
place, at Madam Martine's on Boondael Street in the Ixelles neighborhood.
That was where, whenever he was allowed to, he would sit on the stairs with
nothing to do, no toys to play with and no show of interest from Madam
Martine. He would just sit there and watch the people walking by. One of
the tenants there agreed to open the front door, and to Shaul, it seemed as if
nothing inside had changed since the war, including the stairs that led to the
second floor and the yard by the building. Shaul believed that he lived in the
basement floor, and to his surprise, he found out from Andree that two Jewish
children, brothers, had been hidden with him. Their names were Leon and
Albert Bink. From there, they went to 7 Rue de la Gouttiere, which according
to Andree's notes, he was moved to a year later.

The street was in the center of Brussels, right by a church, and Shaul recalled attending church services and singing psalms in the choir. After returning to Lasne to visit the orphanage, where Shaul and Robert reminisced over fond memories from that period, they continued to Profondsart Castle.

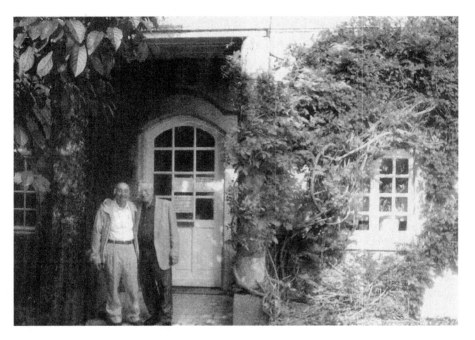

Shaul and Robert on their trip to Lasne

It wasn't easy to find. Most of the people they encountered didn't know it, and only a few people could recall the strange house in the forest where a strange military man now lived. After making their way down a muddy, unpaved path, they saw the castle, which looked like a good setting for a horror movie, with metal turrets and all. The owner of the castle had a limp, probably from his military past, and there was a tatty and faded Belgian flag hanging over one of the windows. To their surprise, he agreed to open the door, which was guarded on both sides by gray stone lions. He led them to the expansive yard that smelled of cat urine. The cats seemed to be the strange man's only friends. The castle, which they remembered as being so full of life, had turned gloomy and dark and the swimming pool was full of dry leaves. Life in winter couldn't have been easy for the children, with the wind blowing wildly and the rain rattling at the windows.

When the left, they saw a strange site: a long table with food at which the strange Belgian military man sat, along with cats on both sides.

2007—THE MOST MOVING CONFERENCE OF ALL

After that visit, and after meeting up with Siegi, the counselor who put a smile back on his face, Shaul finally decided it was time to go back to his past and to tell his story, especially to the younger generations. Wanting to find out more and share the wonderful story of the 3,000 Jewish Belgian children who had survived thanks to the underground movement, motivated him to organize an international conference for all those children hidden in Belgium during the war and to pay tribute to the people who had saved them, Jews and non-Jews alike. Shaul took on the challenging mission and located and invited hundreds of those children to attend the conference.

The conference included talks by psychiatrists, historians and sociologists, and workshops for the hidden children, in which they told each other their stories, sometimes for the very first time in their lives. The guests of honor included Andree Geulen, who was awarded honorary citizenship of Israel by Yad Vashem and appeared on the news on Israeli and Belgian television, surrounded by the dozens of children she had saved. Siegi Hirsch was another guest of honor. The counselor they so loved had become a prominent family therapist in Europe and he also gave a talk, using not only his professional knowledge but also his own personal experience as a concentration camp survivor and counselor to the children now sitting facing him in the hall.

As one could imagine, the air was filled with excitement and sadness, but also with pride. In an instant, decades were peeled away and even the expressions on the participants' faces became childlike and innocent.

The bond shared by the hidden children from Belgium could be felt clearl at the conference. It stemmed from the traumatic loss of contact with thei families, the need to survive and then to integrate into a productive life an to contribute to society. It was a bond that created a special kinship betwee them all.

Shaul stood to the side for a moment and looked at them. To him, the chi dren suddenly looked like a battalion of little soldiers and evoked memorie of the harsh war. Although they weren't together at the time, today they wer discovering all the feelings that they had in common. Suddenly, perhaps fc the first time in his life, Shaul no longer felt alone with his memories.

The fact that there were other children like him, who had similar if not pre cisely the same experiences as he had, evoked a sense of belonging in him an reduced the feelings of loneliness that envelops anyone whose experience trauma on their own, if only just a little.

As a pediatric neurologist and child development specialist, Shaul knew the following facts:

The critical and decisive period in the life of the fetus and then of the chil is from mid-pregnancy to the age of three or four years. It is in those years tha the anatomical structure of the brain is formed: the cells continue to divide a a very quick rate and synaptic connections between the cells are formed wit the help of extensions (axons) that are wrapped in white fat (myeline, whic is important for electric conduction).

Due to the heightened activity of the brain during this period, it is consid ered critical to its proper development. Exposure to potential damage, if to severe, will cause irreparable damage. However, affected areas may still b able to recover, even if they were damaged, because the brain, which is goin through an active process, can utilize other areas that will replace the affecte areas, learn their roles and compensate for the damage caused. This is th flexibility, the plasticity of the brain. This is the period in which motor skill language, cognition, social emotions and the fundamentals of the mental structure develop.

If a child grows up in a loving and supportive environment for the first four, five years of their life, they will be able to develop a basic trust in people, to believe that people are inherently good and can be trusted. But even if a child is hurt during this critical period, they can recover later in ideal environmental conditions for them, and then they can become children who function within the norm.

The professional term for closing these gaps is *catching up*. However, if right from the start, the child is in a hostile and traumatic environment, and remains in that environment past the critical age, there will be cumulative damage, and then the odds of catching up and recovering drop.

Shaul experienced all these theories in practice. To his great luck, he had an excellent start in life. Until the age of five, he was surrounded with the love of his protective parents and family, and also at the end of the war, when he met Siegi Hirsch, his wonderful counselor, who helped him to feel accepted and loved. Because of this, despite the five terrible, lonely, frightening, cold, hungry, affectionless years, and despite the trauma of being suddenly taken from his parents and siblings and coping with life in hiding under a false identity—despite all these—Shaul nevertheless managed to catch up and bridge all the emotional and intellectual gaps.

Talking to and looking at the other hidden children, he could see that most of them had rehabilitated their lives. But unfortunately, he also met and knew quite a few children like him who were less resilient, who couldn't overcome their childhood traumas, who couldn't catch up and recover, and some didn't even start a family. There were children who became psychologically unstable, others became criminals, and some failed to earn an education or learn a profession. And then there was the neighbor's daughter, Irena.

IRENA'S STORY

When Shaul first visited his home at 37a Montenegro Street, his heart was pierced again with the resounding scream that had followed him all his life… the scream of his pregnant neighbor as the Germans dragged her husband away. She was the Czechoslovakian neighbor's wife. The couple emigrated to Belgium in the 1930s, along with their four children. Shaul also remembered playing in the entrance hall of the building with their two younger children, who must have been about his age. When Shaul was preparing for the international hidden children's conference, Regina, his sister, asked him to look for their neighbors, especially Irena, the baby who was born after her father was dragged away. The other children, it turned out, had been taken away and hidden by the underground, whereas the mother had remained alone with the baby. Regina had helped to take care of the baby, had taken her to the family health center, babysat her, fed her and played with her.

With the help of David Inowlocki, the vice president of the Belgian Hidden Children Association, Shaul found the neighbors' sons, who as it turned out, had immigrated to Israel after the war. They told him what had happened to Irena. They, too, were sent to an orphanage sponsored by Dowager Queen Elisabeth, and from there they were sent to the underground. They weren't able to contact her after the war.

Shaul felt that he had to meet Irena. An invisible thread had connected them since that day in 1943, when he was a little boy, horrified by her mother's

358

screams, which still haunted him at night. She was still in her mother's womb, and her fate had already been sealed.

The phone rang for a long time before she answered.

Shaul introduced himself and explained, "I don't know you," he said, "but your mother's screams still echo in my mind."

She immediately started crying and told him about her terrible childhood and youth. The concierge and her husband had hidden her, and when the war ended, they refused to give her to the Jewish institutions. They ran away with her, to the far end of a town called Linkenberg, where they handed her over to the concierge's father and blind mother. It was a desolate place. There was nothing there other than their secluded house, next to a large pit.

She was brought up as a Christian, and she had to do all the housework.

Her "adoptive" family used any excuse to abuse her, both physically and mentally, and she was treated like a slave. She was never sent to school.

After the war, when her brothers could come out of hiding, they tracked her down with the help of a Jewish social worker and went to the secluded house by the abandoned fields. They took a big doll with them. Born in 1942, she was still a little girl and afraid of the people who had taken her in. They were very hostile to her brothers, she refused to go anywhere near them or to take the doll, and so, they immigrated without her to Israel.

At 17, and only after she escaped her terrible life, she married a drunk and lazy man. A few years later, they got divorced, after bringing four children into the world. She brought them up on her own in terrible poverty. Only then did she meet her brothers again and visit them in Israel.

Shaul was shaken to the depths of his soul by her story. He had also suffered terribly, but it was nothing in comparison with Irena's life. After their moving talk, he decided to visit her when they were in Brussels, and he drove to Linkenberg with Dalia and his friend, David Inowlocki.

Irena and her new partner welcomed them warmly. Irena was in her mid-sixties by then, short with bright blue eyes, and they could see how beautiful she must have been when she was younger. Her current partner was 92 years old, 28 years her senior. He was a single Jewish artist who, during World War II, had escaped to the Belgian Congo. Years later, when he returned, he found Irena. Despite the big age difference between them, they obviously loved each other. Shaul, Dalia and David met them in the entrance, because their apartment, if you could call it that, was a tiny room the size of a kitchen, which served as both a living room and a kitchen, and there was a small bedroom nook leading off from it. The walls were covered with her husband's countless bright, sensual paintings with a clear African influence. Although it was small and they were poor, Irena had undoubtedly found the love of her life and peace of mind, after the many years of turmoil and suffering.

COMMEMORATION ACTIVITIES

After the Belgian hidden children's conference, Shaul got swept up in activities to commemorate the wondrous story of how it all happened. He realized that although the story may be well known in Belgium, it certainly wasn't known elsewhere, including in Israel.

People from Belgian television came with the director Bernard Balteau to the conference in Jerusalem, and they helped to spread the story in Belgium. Balteau painstakingly filmed the entire conference, including the lectures and discussions, and he and Shaul clicked immediately.

Bernard Balteau was of Walloon descent and had worked in Belgian television for years as a documentary director. After he made the film about Andree Geulen, he grew close to the Jewish community. So much so, that he fell in love with Jewish humor and loved Jewish jokes, particularly when Siegi Hirsch was telling them. After the conference, the two decided that the discourse on the Belgian hidden children should continue and that their story should be commemorated through a documentary. Shaul's aim was to tell the heroic story of the underground's part in hiding the children, while highlighting the heroic women who were part of the rescue team.

To Shaul's great surprise, Belgian television agreed to help by covering Balteau's expenses. But they had one condition that Shaul found hard to accept: the film would tell the story of the hidden children through one, personal story. They chose Shaul as the film's lead character. This may have been because his story of resilience covered two periods, the Holocaust, and immigration to Israel.

In the first phase, in November 2007, a short workshop was organized in the Ardennes and it was attended by several hidden children, Andree Geulen, Siegi Hirsch and Tali and Ronit—Shaul and Dalia's daughters, who represented the second generation. During the workshop, they discussed the mechanism of repression and denial that served the hidden children for years and their sudden awakening when they were older and ready to explore their past. Balteau took advantage of Tali and Ronit's participation to film material for the documentary. They visited Shaul's childhood family home, the two houses where Shaul was hidden during the war, the Holocaust Museum at the Mechelen transit camp, and Andree Geulen at her home, where they had an emotional reunion. At the end of their stay, they happened to learn that it was the last day of a traveling exhibition of photos of Jews who'd been sent on Transport No. 20. It was on the outskirts of Antwerp. They hurried to the exhibition, where they found pictures of Shaul's parents. Unaware of the cameras, Tali and Shaul's reactions were filmed without them knowing and the footage brought the film to an emotional close. The random manner in which it was filmed gave it an authentic and natural feel, and they didn't stage a single scene.

Filming continued in June 2008, and this time Shaul visited the children's home in Lasne with Siegi and Robert Fuks. A month later, Balteau came to Israel and they visited Nitzanim, Aloney Yitzchak and Dana-Dwek Children's Hospital at the Tel Aviv Medical Center. All that time, there was still no producer or funding for the film. The film was up in the air and they weren't at all sure that it would happen. But Shaul didn't give up. Through a Jewish member of the Belgian parliament, he contacted the Dardenne brothers, who were directors and producers with an excellent reputation (and films that excelled in their minimalistic and intimate atmosphere). There was even a trend named after them: Dardennism. They've won four Cannes Golden Palm Awards in a variety of categories and have been nominated in many competitions. The Dardenne brothers were friendly and modest, and their name opened doors for funding and producing the film. Also, the brothers' contribution to the editing, design and atmosphere of the film was crucial. They decided to call the film *Les Enfants Sans Ombre (Children Without a Shadow)*. *That was a* term that Siegi Hirsch used in the film because it's a story about a child, or children, who had lost their shadow during the war...their family, history, name, language, and had then learned to form a new shadow during the process of surviving, recovering, and creating new lives for themselves.

In October 2009, they had two screenings of the film, one at Yad Vashem in Jerusalem, and the other at the Museum of the Jewish People at Beit Hatfutsot in Tel Aviv. The film was later screened on Holocaust Remembrance Day on Israeli Channel 10 and in the three cinematheques, in Tel Aviv, Jerusalem and Haifa. At the same time, it was screened a number of times on Belgian television, at the Shoah Memorial in Paris, on International Holocaust Remembrance Day in London, Canada and the U.S. (three times in New York and once in L.A.).

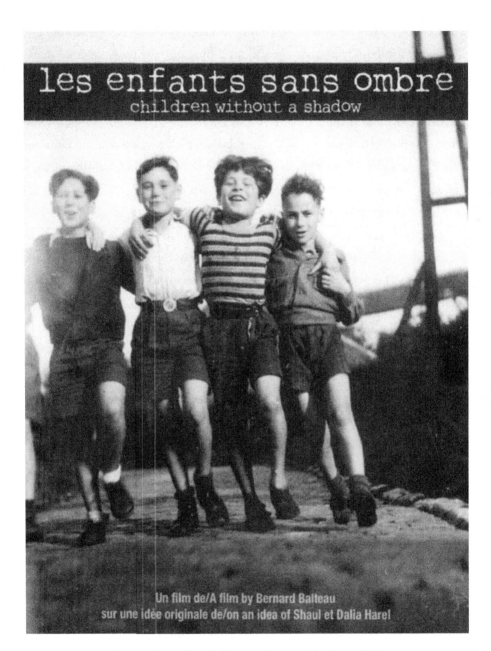

les enfants sans ombre
children without a shadow

Un film de/A film by Bernard Balteau
sur une idée originale de/on an idea of Shaul et Dalia Harel

Cover of the film Children without a Shadow, 2009

Every year, Shaul is invited to screen the film in various places around Israel, and he sees this as an important mission. Like many of the hidden children, he is close to 84-years-old, and he's afraid that the generation will soon die out and there'll be no one left to tell their story. He considers his three children's and even his grandchildren's involvement as an achievement and he knows not to take it for granted.

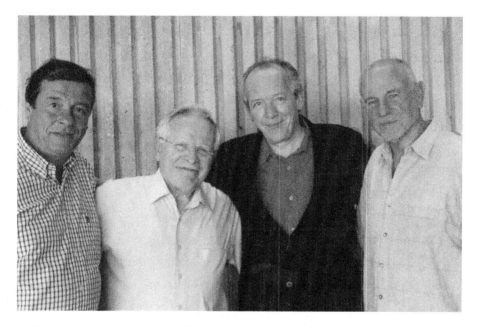

From left to right— Bernard Balteau, Shaul, Luc Dardenne and Judd Ne'eman outside the film screening in 2009

He therefore continued his commemorative work and to pay tribute to the people who had played such an important role. In September 2011, Andree Geulen turned 90, and it was 20 years since the Belgian Hidden Children Association was founded. A special event was planned to be held in Belgium.

Shaul had no idea how to express his admiration and appreciation to Andree, after years of learning to love her sensitivity, wit and love of life.

It was dusk at a hotel on the Dead Sea, before an opera performance at the foot of Masada, when Shaul decided to go soak in the hot tub and relax. He was still trying to decide what gift to give Andree. After all, she had everything: a loving and dedicated family, she was surrounded by the children she helped to hide, who would visit her from time to time, and her standard of living was fine. He remembered her life story and the captivating stories that filled it. Suddenly, as he got into the hot tub, like Archimedes who found inspiration in the bath, he felt the words he wanted to say about Andree Geulen flow from his memory. He ran to their hotel room, asked Dalia to bring paper and a pencil, and he started reciting Andrea's story to her, one stanza after another.

Dalia couldn't believe her ears. Shaul had never written a poem like that for her; he had always been a bit closed and reserved. She put all his words to paper and then worked on rhyming them. But Shaul had greater aspirations. He decided to turn the poem into a song. First, he asked their friend Keren Hadar to sing it. Then he appealed to the composer Rafi Kadishzon, who with the generous help of Dan Almagor (who knew just how to match the words to the music) the musical poem "Mademoiselle" was born.

The first time that Dalia and Shaul heard Keren sing the song, they knew it would be a hit. The words and melody were profoundly moving and touching. It took a lot of effort to produce the song and record it, but it all paid off when the audience in Belgium heard the song, which had French and English subtitles, and they saw many people wiping away a tear, including the Belgian ambassador to Israel and her husband.

The song was uploaded to YouTube and had more than 250,000 views around the world, especially in the U.S.

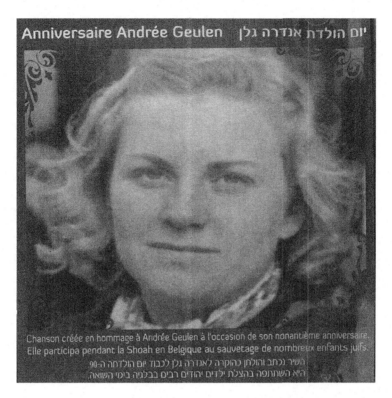

Anniversaire Andrée Geulen | יום הולדת אנדרה גלן

Chanson créée en hommage à Andrée Geulen à l'occasion de son nonantième anniversaire. Elle participa pendant la Shoah en Belgique au sauvetage de nombreux enfants juifs.

השיר נכתב והולחן כהוקרה לאנדרה גלן לכבוד יום הולדתה ה-90. היא השתתפה בהצלת ילדים יהודים רבים בבלגיה בימי השואה.

The cover of the "Mademoiselle" recording

They still weren't done. When Siegi Hirsch turned 90, Shaul decided that the nicest tribute he could make would be with words and music.

This time, he wrote the song in French and Roni Porat, the well-known composer and conductor, produced it. The production process was even more complex than producing "Mademoiselle," with nine musicians, three young background singers and the vocalist Emmanuel Hannoun.

The song described the special bond between Shaul and Siegi, who had a great impact on him and brought the smile back to his face, that memorable year at the orphanage in Lasne, and their unforgettable reunion 60 years later, when they discovered that the murderous doctor who had starved Shaul's brother to death had also, on a whim, granted Siegi his life back.

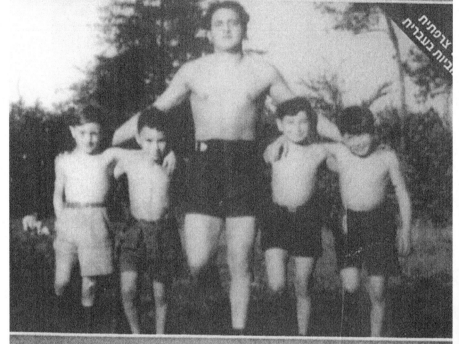

Anniversaire de Siegi Hirsch

עמותת בוצרת
אופריה

Chanson créée en hommage à Siegi Hirsch à l'occasion de son 90ème anniversaire.

Le moniteur qui a rendu le sourire à de nombreux enfants juifs après la Shoah en Belgique

The tape cover of the song about Siegi for his 90th birthday

The tape was played at a seminar on resilience in Brussels, in honor of Siegi on his 90th birthday. Top experts on the subject participated. The song touched the hearts of them all.

Another conference, *Resilience in Action: Special Colloquium on Trauma and Resilience in Children During and After the Holocaust,* was held on International Holocaust Remembrance Day in 2016. It was attended by the German ambassador to Israel, the Ra'anana Symphonette Orchestra, and children's choir performed the song.

All these activities on the Holocaust and resilience opened up a new field for Shaul, in addition to his clinical and research work, and it gives him a great sense of satisfaction.

At the end of 2015, Shaul received the King Leopold medal of honor for his work on commemorating the courage of and part played by the Belgians in hiding children, and for strengthening the relationship between Israel and Belgium. The ceremony was held at the house of the Belgian ambassador to Israel, where the Belgian Foreign Minister and Deputy Prime Minister, Diedier Reynders, gave Shaul the award.

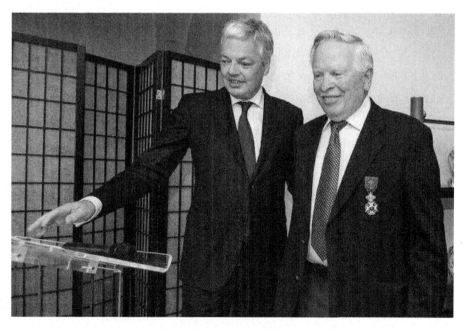

Shaul with the Belgian Foreign Minister and Deputy Prime Minister,
Mr. Didier Reynders

EPILOGUE – I BELIEVE

This book is not intended to be an orderly, chronological autobiography. It is an expression of my desire to share with the reader the experiences, both negative and positive, that shaped my life. The book reviews my family background, our exodus to France, the Holocaust in Belgium, my immigration to and integration in Israel, establishing a family, my studies, and medical career in pediatric neurology and child development.

This book describes a life course that is a kind of a Belgian-Israeli saga, leading from the loss of my first shadow in life as a result of the circumstances I found myself in, to forming a new shadow.

Luckily, for the first five years of my life, I got to live with a warm and loving family, which instilled confidence in me and gave me a basic sense of security for the rest of my journey. The Holocaust was traumatic and painful for me, when at about the age of five, I had to say a final goodbye to my parents, my brother Marcel, and my sister Tola. Most of the memories were erased from my mind, and I was left with only flashbacks. I had to dig deep into my memory and try to separate imagination from truth, and perhaps that is what's interesting in my life story. I asked my sister Regina to help me, as she was nine years older than me. She was with me at the beginning of that period, and being 14 years old, her memories of that period were deeply ingrained in her.

Although the ability to repress my memories allowed me and others to build a new life, most of the hidden children were left with scars…a scratch on the fabric of our lives. We tried to cover it under different shades of camouflage, but the scratch is still there, and we have to cope with it. Whenever I look at my youngest grandchildren, six, seven and eight years old, I have nightmares that if I hadn't been hidden by those brave people in Belgium, my short life would have certainly ended in the ovens in Auschwitz, and I remember the startling statistic that *not a single child under the age of 13 who was sent to Auschwitz from Mechelen survived.*

Siegi Hirsch, our legendary counselor and mentor and a survivor of Auschwitz himself, called us *children without a shadow* or *the children of silence...* children who could cry without making a sound, without shedding a tear.

We repressed our fears and our troubles, and created a new, joyful world with Siegi, one of play and laughter, filled with stories and jokes, and sometimes, with tragic Jewish tragedy. Siegi claimed that we got used to negotiating with life and survival at an early age. Only after many years, when I grew stronger, did I begin to understand the course of my life.

My friend, Boris Cyrulnik, a well-known psychiatrist and a hidden child himself, became the expert on resilience and published many books on the subject. He wrote, that today, Lot's wife could turn back today and look at her past, and continue on the path to happiness, without fear of turning into a pillar of salt. As such, he claimed, survival is not just resilience, but also the ability to learn to live.

For me, the real heroes of the Holocaust in Belgium were the rescuers, particularly the 12 women and two men, including the marvelous women who saved me, Andree Geulen and Ida Sterno, who all risked their lives to save around 3,000 Jewish children.

In my opinion, there are other heroes whose importance is not stressed enough, and they are the parents who knowingly had the courage to say goodbye to their children, often forever, in order to save them from the clutches of the Nazis.

For the mothers, it was like the judgement of Solomon. This story of rescue

371

and survival proves that the values of humanism didn't disappear when faced with the Nazis' barbarism.

It's easy to think that the hidden children's story ended happily. After all, they survived and went on to build new lives. But their victory was not absolute. The impact of what they were deprived of and of their losses, with entire chapters deleted from their childhood, cannot be estimated. I often wonder, mostly when I'm watching my youngest grandchildren, and unlike in the past, when I watched my own children and my older grandchildren, and I see them so happy and enveloped in warmth and love, how I felt when I was suddenly and so cruelly taken away from my parents and siblings to the chilly hiding places, and the moves that followed. Luckily, I don't seem to remember. But I never forget the fact that more than 5,000 Jewish children in Belgium were murdered by the Nazis, and that some of the survivors were not resilient and found life hard to navigate. What a loss to the families and to society.

As an expert on child development, I always point out the importance of early childhood and the neurobiological principle of continuous and cumulative damage to the brain. The more children suffer at an early age from sequential damages, the lower their chances of recovery, especially when the environment they land up in continues to be traumatic and harmful. I, too, suffered from a sequence of damages, during the Holocaust and while trying to integrate in Israel. But I was fortunate to land up at Alonei Yitzchak with the Youth Aliya movement, which gave me the opportunity I needed to be rehabilitated, and to integrate into Israeli life. This fact contains a universal message, as even today, the world is filled with children who are being traumatized or hidden and are suffering from cumulative damage caused by terrorism, hunger, bombing and shelling, or the loss of their close families. The enlightened world has got to make sure that they survive and recover, and that they don't suffer from physical and mental damage for the rest of their lives.

I look back on my relatively long life and believe that my most important work was creating a loving family. My wife Dalia has supported me all the way, my children have a close relationship that makes my heart swell. For me, living in Israel and starting a family is the best answer to the Nazi plot to wipe out the Jewish people. Plus, I was blessed with a life rich in fascinating and exciting events, in achieving, and in having my achievements recognized. I therefore decided to share these experiences and memories with readers other than my family and close friends. I hope that the universally humane and optimistic messages expressed in this book have some kind of impact.

If this book can lead young people to fulfill their dreams, against all odds, that's good enough for me.

Shaul Harel, *April 2021*

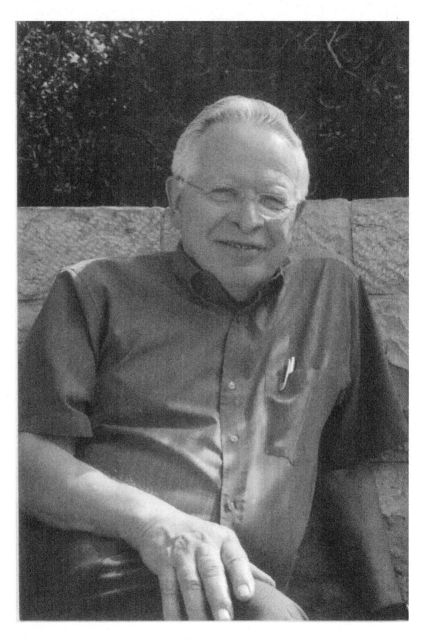

Shaul Harel

ACKNOWLEDGEMENTS

My heartfelt thanks to Ela Moskovits-Weiss for joining us in writing this book and for the contribution of her creative and moving writing talent.

Special thanks to my wife Dalia, whose dedication and perseverance, precision and thoroughness, provided the factual infrastructure for my book, and participated in writing the book while adding a humorous touch.

I also thank Steimatzky Publishing and its management, in particular the Director of Publishing, Evelyn Levy, who found my stories interesting, encouraged us and supported us throughout the process. By so doing, she allowed me to fulfill my dream and expose readers to the story of my life, the life of a hidden child surviving the Holocaust in Belgium, a life that is interwoven with the history of Israel.

A LIST OF BOOKS I FOUND HELPFUL

Raul Hilberg. *The Destruction of the European Jews—Belgium*, Hebrew edition, Yad Vashem and the Ben Gurion University, 2012.

Saul Friedländer. *The Years of Extermination: Nazi Germany and the Jews, 1939-1945*, Hebrew edition, Am Oved, 2009.

Yisrael Gutman and Michael Berenbaum, editors. *Anatomy of the Auschwitz Death Camp*, Hebrew edition, Yad Vashem, 2003

Jim Baggot. *Atomic: The First War of Physics and the Secret History of the Atom Bomb 1939-49*, Hebrew edition, Books in the Attic, Yedioth Aharonot-Sifrei Hemed, 2012.

Sylvain Brachfeld. *A Gift of Life: The Deportation and the Rescue of the Jews in Occupied Belgium (1940-1944)*, Hebrew edition, Yedioth Aharonot-Sifrei Hemed, 2000

Boris Cyrulnik. *Sauve–Toi la vie t'appelle Odile Jacob*, Paris, 2012.

Alain van Crugten. *Pourquoi Pas Moi (Temoignage de Robert Fuks, Enfant Cache)*, Averbode 2006.

Printed in Great Britain
by Amazon